European School of Oncology

Monographs

Series Editor: U. Veronesi

The European School of Oncology gratefully acknowledges
sponsorship for the Task Force received from
ZENECA Pharmaceuticals

Springer
Berlin
Heidelberg
New York
Barcelona
Budapest
Hong Kong
London
Milan
Paris
Santa Clara
Singapore
Tokyo

L. Denis (Ed.)

Antiandrogens in Prostate Cancer

A Key to Tailored Endocrine Treatment

With 54 Figures and 39 Tables

Springer

Professor Dr. Louis Denis

Vrije Universiteit Brussel
Oncologisch Centrum Antwerpen
Algemeen Ziekenhuis Middelheim
Lindendreef 1
2020 Antwerp, Belgium

ISBN-13: 978-3-642-45747-0 e-ISBN-13: 978-3-642-45745-6
DOI: 10.1007/978-3-642-45745-6

Library of Congress Cataloging-in-Publication Data
Antiandrogens in prostate cancer / L. Denis, (ed.).
(ESO monographs)
Includes bibliographical references.
ISBN 978-3-642-45747-0
1. Prostate--Cancer--Chemotherapy. 2. Antiandrogens--Therapeutic use. I. Denis, L. II. Series: Monographs (European School of Oncology)
RC280.P7A58 1996 616.99'463--dc20

Softcover reprint of the hardcover 1st edition 1996

Typesetting: Camera ready by editor
Printed on acid-free paper

Foreword

The European School of Oncology came into existence to respond to a need for information, education and training in the field of the diagnosis and treatment of cancer. There are two main reasons why such an initiative was considered necessary. Firstly, the teaching of oncology requires a rigorously multidisciplinary approach which is difficult for the Universities to put into practice since their system is mainly disciplinary orientated. Secondly, the rate of technological development that impinges on the diagnosis and treatment of cancer has been so rapid that it is not an easy task for medical faculties to adapt their curricula flexibly.

With its residential courses for organ pathologies and the seminars on new techniques (laser, monoclonal antibodies, imaging techniques etc.) or on the principal therapeutic controversies (conservative or mutilating surgery, primary or adjuvant chemotherapy, radiotherapy alone or integrated), it is the ambition of the European School of Oncology to fill a cultural and scientific gap and, thereby, create a bridge between the University and Industry and between these two and daily medical practice.

One of the more recent initiatives of ESO has been the institution of permanent study groups, also called task forces, where a limited number of leading experts are invited to meet once a year with the aim of defining the state of the art and possibly reaching a consensus on future developments in specific fields of oncology.

The ESO Monograph series was designed with the specific purpose of disseminating the results of these study group meetings, and providing concise and updated reviews of the topic discussed.

It was decided to keep the layout relatively simple, in order to restrict the costs and make the monographs available in the shortest possible time, thus overcoming a common problem in medical literature: that of the material being outdated even before publication.

Umberto Veronesi
Chairman Scientific Committee
European School of Oncology

Contents

Introduction

Louis Denis

Oncological Centre Antwerp, Department of Urology, A.Z. Middelheim, Lindendreef 1, Antwerp 2020, Belgium

The European School of Oncology Task Force meeting on antiandrogens was arranged to create a forum for discussion between clinicians, experts in the field of prostate cancer, and scientists with a particular, specialised understanding of the endocrinology and biochemistry relevant to the use of these drugs. The aim of the meeting was to focus attention on the current knowledge regarding the mode of action of the antiandrogens and their use in the management of the disease. The timing of the meeting was most appropriate, with the clinician facing important advances in the knowledge of prostate cancer, associated with a wider range of treatment options, but at the same time much aware of the lack of change over the past few decades in patient mortality.

In many parts of the world this unacceptable state of affairs has led to exciting new screening initiatives to search for localised disease, while in other regions it has resulted in attempts to offer earlier treatment. Despite a certain degree of success in approximately 50% of patients, the lead-time bias merely delays the necessity of treating large numbers of the remaining patients presenting with advanced disease by the year 2000.

As Peter Boyle stated in our previous ESO Monograph, "Prostate Cancer 2000", the ageing population of the European Union will provide a strong determinant in the consideration of prostatic cancer as an endemic disease in its member states.

The systemic nature of this disease at the advanced stage directs the attention to global therapeutic strategies, where endpoints of treatment outcome such as survival, progression, quality of life and the costs of treatment are important policy points for any future health care programme.

The antiandrogens play a key role in some of the important questions facing the investigator and clinician alike. The question as to whether there is a better antiandrogen must be posed. The precise clinical indications for antiandrogen therapy, whether as monotherapy or in combination, must be addressed. We cannot state that there is a particular therapeutic option for the individual patient, but we do wish to present all the appropriate facts in such a way that discerning readers have guidance allowing treatment to be tailored to a particular patient.

It is our privilege to thank the faculty, not only for their enthusiasm and dedication, but also for their patience, which has allowed them to come to terms with a divergent array of options and convictions that emanated from the group. We are grateful to the laboratory scientists, Griffiths, Neumann, Neri, Furr and Gaillard and to our clinical experts, Schröder, Labrie, Blackledge and Mahler. We also appreciated the expert guidance in our discussions of Professor F. Rocco of the European Institute of Oncology. As always, we are pleased to express our gratitude to Mrs. Rita Denie of the Oncological Centre of Antwerp for her immaculate secretarial assistance and to the European School of Oncology team and its director, Dr. A. Costa, for their support.

The completion of this manuscript would have been impossible without the expertise and patience of Ms Marije de Jager of ESO and Ms Barbara Montenbruck of Springer Verlag.

Some Aspects of the Molecular Endocrinology of Prostatic Cancer

K. Griffiths, C.L. Eaton, M.E. Harper, A.M.K. Weir and B.A.J. Evans

Tenovus Cancer Research Centre, University of Wales College of Medicine, Heath Park, Cardiff, Wales CF4 4XX, United Kingdom

A recent report from the World Health Organisation [1] reveals that carcinoma of the prostate is the second most commonly diagnosed cancer after skin cancer in the male population of the United States of America and the second most common cause of death from cancer after that of lung. The age-adjusted mortality rates per 100,000 vary in different regions of the United States from 18.9 for white males in Arkansas to 55.5 for black men in North Carolina, probably the highest mortality rate in the world [2]. Overall around the world, the incidence of prostatic cancer is increasing at an annual rate of approximately 2% to 3% (Fig. 1), with the lifetime risk of the disease developing in North American men being nearly 10% [3].

Prostatic cancer and benign prostatic hyperplasia (BPH) are conditions that rarely present in men under the age of 50 years. Moreover, the prevalence of both symptomatic clinical BPH, often with bladder outflow obstruction, and cancer increases with advancing years. With an ever increasing proportion of the population in the developing countries over the age of 65 years, prostatic disease, both BPH and cancer, are becoming major public health problems [4]. Prostatectomy for the treatment of bladder outflow obstruction is the second most common surgical procedure undergone by males worldwide. The lifetime risk of a man of 40 in the United States undergoing a prostatectomy, 10% in 1968 [5], is now reported to be more than 30% [6].

It is very appropriate that there is a continual reassessment of our understanding of the natural history of both prostatic cancer and BPH, and of the molecular processes that may exercise a role in the pathogenesis of these diseases. There are fundamental issues to be addressed, one in particular being the influence of race and geographical variation on the worldwide incidence of prostatic cancer [2], as the disease is rarely seen in the Asian people of, for example, Thailand, China or Japan [7]. The age-adjusted incidence rates in the United States are more than 30 times that in Japan and studies of migrant populations strongly suggest that certain dietary components in the Asian diet may well influence the aetiology of the disease [8]. The mortality rate of prostatic cancer increases to at least half that of the indigenous American men for those Japanese migrants who settle in North America.

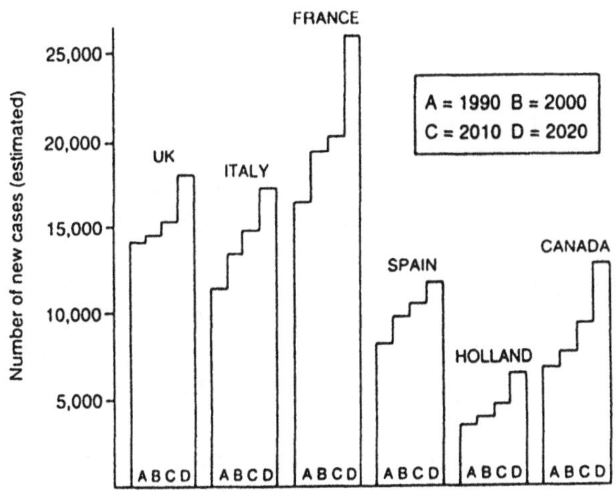

Fig. 1. Diagrammatic representation of the estimated increase in the incidence of cancer of the prostate over the next 3 decades. Data from P. Boyle [3]

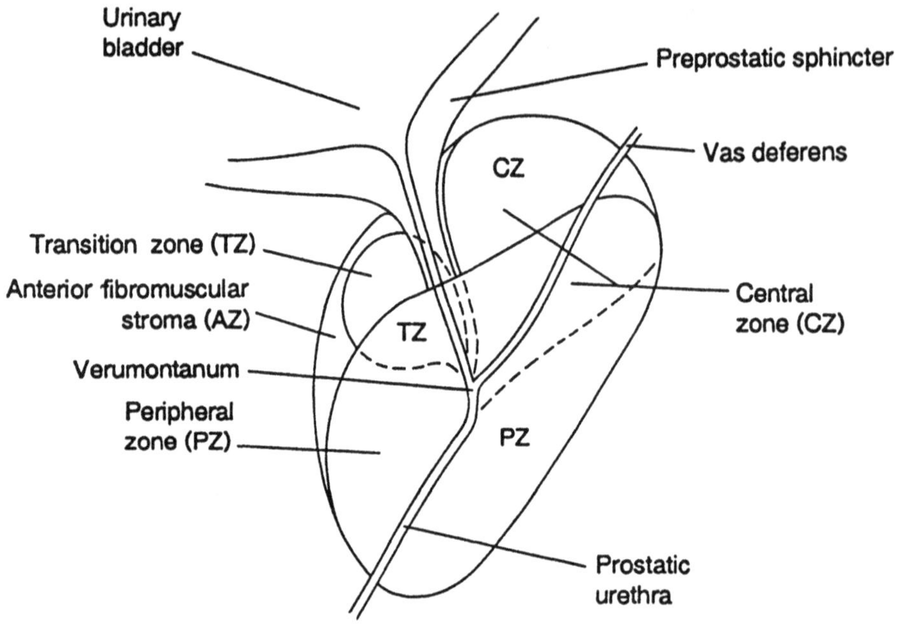

Fig. 2. The zonal anatomy of the prostate gland. From J. McNeal [9]

Intraprostatic Origins of Cancer

Another fundamental issue to be considered relates to the previously held belief [9] that the major proportion of prostatic cancer originated in the peripheral zone of the gland (Fig. 2), with the transition zone the site of origin of BPH. Despite controversy [10,11], the general consensus amongst urologists was that the two conditions were not directly related but represented independent disorders, and by inference their aetiologies were considered distinct. Recent reports [12] indicate, however, that although 70% of cancers do originate in the peripheral zone, approximately 25% develop in the centrally located transition zone and are identified as "incidental carcinoma" in transurethrally resected tissue removed at prostatectomy (TURP) for BPH. Although once considered of low malignant potential, detailed morphological study [13] of these T1 cancers reveals a range of volume and grade not dissimilar from T2 cancer, thereby providing little support for the concept that they are intrinsically different from the latter, which develop in the peripheral zone, close to the rectal surface, and can be recognised at digital rectal examination.

Is BPH therefore causally related to prostatic cancer? Clearly with certain features common to both, it is not unreasonable to reconsider the question and a recent, more rigorous re-evaluation of the pathology and epidemiology of prostate disease does suggest a potential relationship between the transition zone cancer and BPH [12]. Both diseases show an increasing incidence with ageing, have related natural histories and are androgen-associated conditions that respond to androgen withdrawal therapy: cancer is found incidentally in up to 10% of TURP specimens, with an incidence which is age dependent, and neither BPH nor cancer develop in men castrated early in life.

Tissue resected at prostatectomy for BPH contains lesions resembling low grade acinar carcinoma referred to as atypical adenomatous hyperplasia (AAH) [14], which in some ways may be analogous to another lesion, prostatic intraepithelial neoplasia (PIN), identified in the peripheral zone and considered a premalignant lesion. Both should probably be recognised as premalignant lesions [15,16], i.e., early stages in the escape of epithelial cell proliferation from growth regulation. The prevalence and grade of AAH and PIN are greater in prostates with carcinoma than in those without [17,18]. Little is known about the natural history of prostatic cancer, nor about the relationship of AAH and PIN to the clinically asymptomatic "latent carcinoma" present in 30% of prostates of men over 50 years of age [19] and in men of all races from East and West [20]. Progressive disease has been reported in 33% of stage T1b cancer patients within 4 years (Fig. 3) [21], a frequency higher than that of stage T2a cancer, palpated rectally [22]: the low-volume,

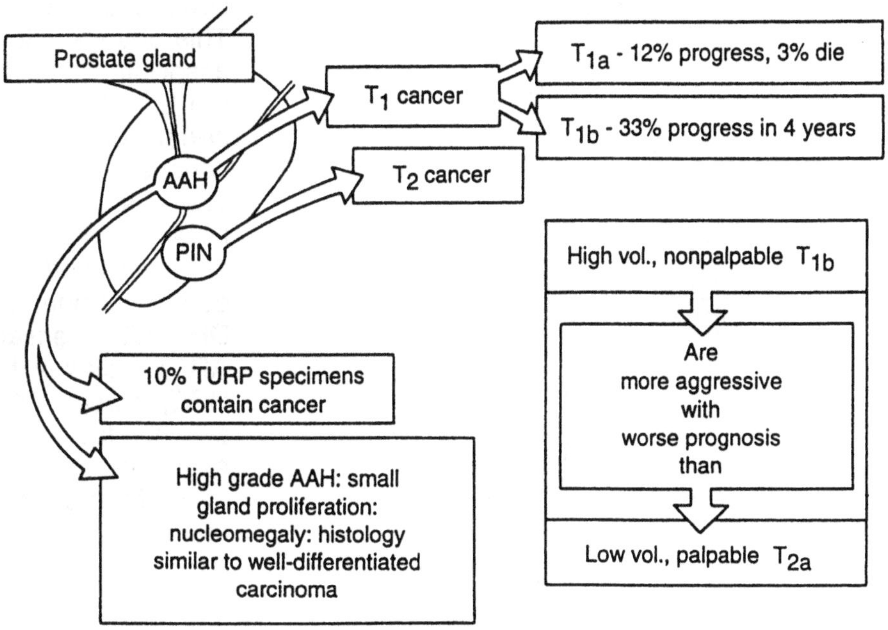

Fig. 3. The localisation of premalignant lesions of the prostate with simple illustration of the progression of early foci of cancer

differentiated T1a cancer does not always have a low malignant propensity [23,24].

Although prostatic cancer is a disease which presents in later years, its origins may well have been present many years earlier, and more information is needed on the molecular events involved in the initiation of AAH and PIN, their progression to focal cancer and the development of the slowly growing latent cancer to the aggressive malignant phenotype.

Androgens and Prostatic Cancer

The scientific studies of Charles Huggins first established the androgen-responsive nature of prostatic cancer and provided the scientific basis for the treatment of metastatic disease by androgen-ablative therapy [25,26]. It was the conviction of Huggins [27] that the slow but consistent rate of growth of prostatic cancer was determined by a balance between the effects of intraprostatic factors and other growth-restraining components of the "soil" in which the tumour resided, a concept much in line with modern thoughts on the processes of carcinogenesis [28,29]. The clinical behaviour of prostatic cancer reflects androgen responsiveness, and first-line endocrine therapy such as orchidectomy or the administration of LHRH analogues is effective in the short term. Of patients with metastatic disease, 70-80% experience subjective symptomatic relief and 40-60% achieve objective remission after androgen withdrawal [30], although the treatment is palliative and relapse generally occurs within 1 to 2 years, disease progression being seen as the autonomous proliferation of hormone-insensitive clones of cancer cells.

Androgens are clearly essential for the normal growth of the prostate gland. Earlier studies [31] demonstrated the rapid growth phase of the prostate from the time of adolescence to the early 20s, when the gland attains the adult maximal size. The increased rate of growth observed after the age of 50 relates to the development of clinical BPH in later years. Of particular interest, however, is the increasing prevalence of microscopic BPH, areas of epithelial hyperplasia, with increasing age from the early 20s. This process of marked cellular proliferation is recognised in men of all races from both East and West [31], although the incidence of clinical BPH in Asia is less than that in the western countries [32]. The fact that the prevalent latent cancer [20] rarely develops into malignant prostatic disease in the oriental man also deserves some consideration [2,7].

Within the prostate gland, testosterone, the principal plasma androgen, is converted to 5α-dihydrotestosterone (DHT) by the 5α-reductase enzyme system localised on the nuclear membrane. DHT preferentially binds to the androgen receptor (AR) in the target cells (Fig. 4), 5 times more avidly than does testosterone.

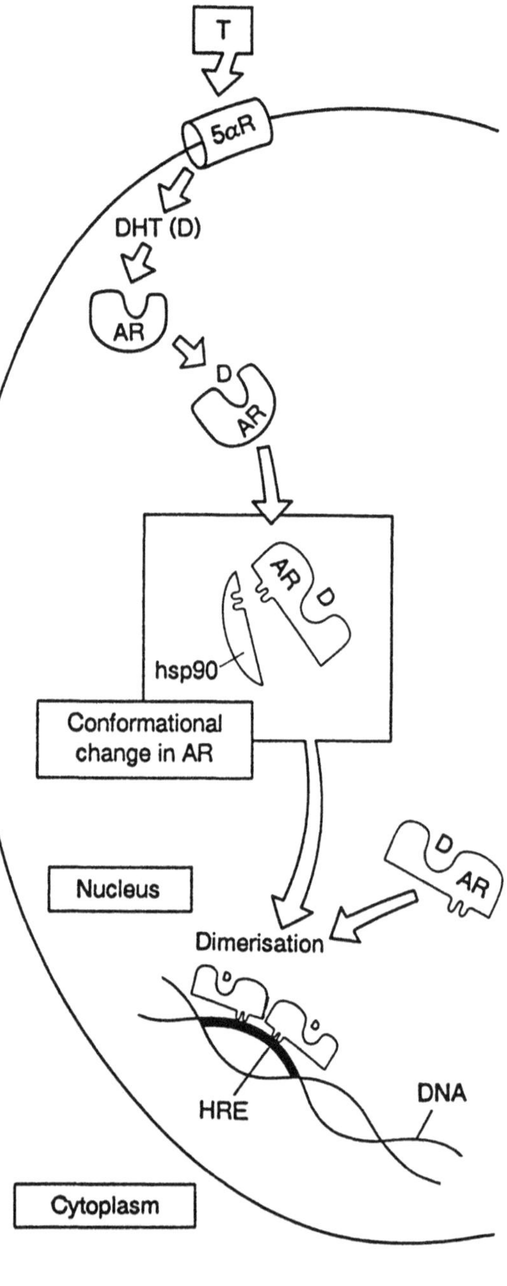

Fig. 4. Simple representation of the processes by which DHT is formed from testosterone, binds to AR and, as a DHT-AR complex, associates with hormone response elements in the form of dimers

The formation of the DHT-AR complex is of paramount importance in the activation not only of the growth regulatory pathways, but also of the processes involved in the synthesis and secretion of the secretory proteins such as prostate-specific antigen (PSA). The DHT-AR complex modulates gene expression in the prostate gland, the binding of DHT to AR "triggering" a conformational change, unmasking the DNA binding domain of the receptor protein. This change allows the DHT-AR complex to associate with specific recognition sequences, the hormone response elements (HRE), upstream of the transcription start sites of the various androgen-responsive genes.

There is evidence that the unmasking of the DNA binding domain relates to the release of the associated heat shock protein 90 (hsp90), conformational changes [33-36] that allow DHT-AR dimerisation [37]. The activated DHT-AR complexes bind as homodimers to the HRE, thereby acting as ligand-dependent transcription factors associating with the enhancer sequences on the genome to modulate the activity of the androgen-responsive genes. DHT therefore exercises a pivotal role in the growth regulatory processes, with the prostate gland failing to grow in the absence of DHT and neither BPH nor cancer developing in men castrated early in life. Studies show that the gland does not grow in men from the Dominican Republic with an inherited 5α-reductase deficiency causing male pseudohermaphroditism [38]. Such men develop reasonable musculature at puberty, manifest relatively normal genitalia, libido and erections, presumably the biological effects of testosterone, but the prostate is either absent or remains vestigial in the absence of DHT.

The processes by which DHT influences prostatic growth are now becoming better understood [39]. Castration causes a reduction in prostate size with a rapid decrease in cell number and DNA content to 10% of normal by 10 days post-castration, the surviving cells presumably being the stem cells [40,41]. Administration of androgen causes cell proliferation and the restoration of cell number, but exogenous androgen does not cause prostatic overgrowth, the gland merely attaining the maximal adult size. After androgen administration, there is a lag period of 24-48 hours before an increase in DNA synthesis can be recognised, with the level peaking between 72-96 hours before the cell number is restored. Castration and the depletion of intraprostatic AR instigate prostatic involution, and after androgen administration reaccumulation of AR "switches on" the processes involved in cellular proliferation (Fig. 5). The increase in nuclear AR, however, precedes DNA synthesis by many hours [41], a finding which indicates that androgens are essential, but not directly responsible, for cell proliferation, and that the intercession of other intermediary growth regulatory factors is necessary.

The DHT-AR complexes associate as homodimers (Fig. 4) and with high affinity to the HREs, a process that is facilitated by the particular symmetry of the nucleotide sequences of the HRE and either promotes or suppresses gene transcription (Fig. 6). The promoter region, the nucleotide sequences at the 5' upstream end of the gene, is concerned with gene regulation. This can either involve transcription initiation, or the promoter region can influence the rate of gene transcription; the latter process is more often mediated by specific DNA binding proteins such as DHT-AR, regulatory transacting modulators that would include other protein transcription factors which could promote or restrain gene expression. It could be envisaged that the modulating effect of the DHT-AR complexes is to influence the spatial orientation of the DNA strands such that the change facilitates the access of the transcription factors to the nucleotide sequences. The regulation of gene transcription by steroid hormones is the topic of many excellent reviews [42-45], but the interaction between steroid receptors, other transcription factors and DNA is discussed in a later section of this chapter.

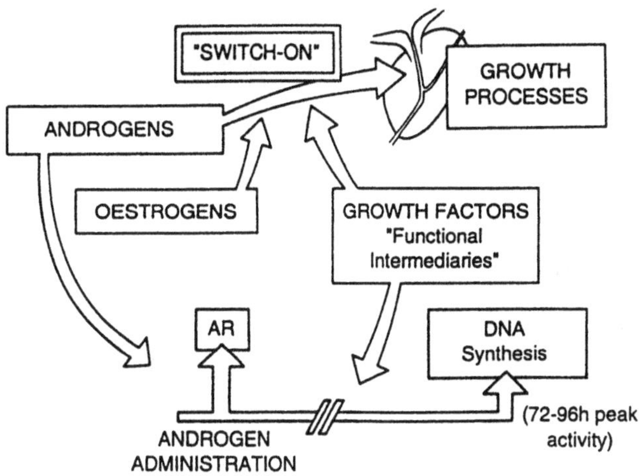

Fig. 5. Androgens "switch on" growth processes, but other intermediary growth regulatory factors are more directly implicated in promoting cell proliferation and DNA synthesis

Growth Regulatory Factors

The presence of testes and an ageing factor would appear to be two principal parameters that relate to the aetiology of BPH and prostatic cancer [46]. Since neither condition develops in men castrated prior to puberty, androgens, but more specifically DHT, would seem to be implicated in the pathogenesis of prostate disease.

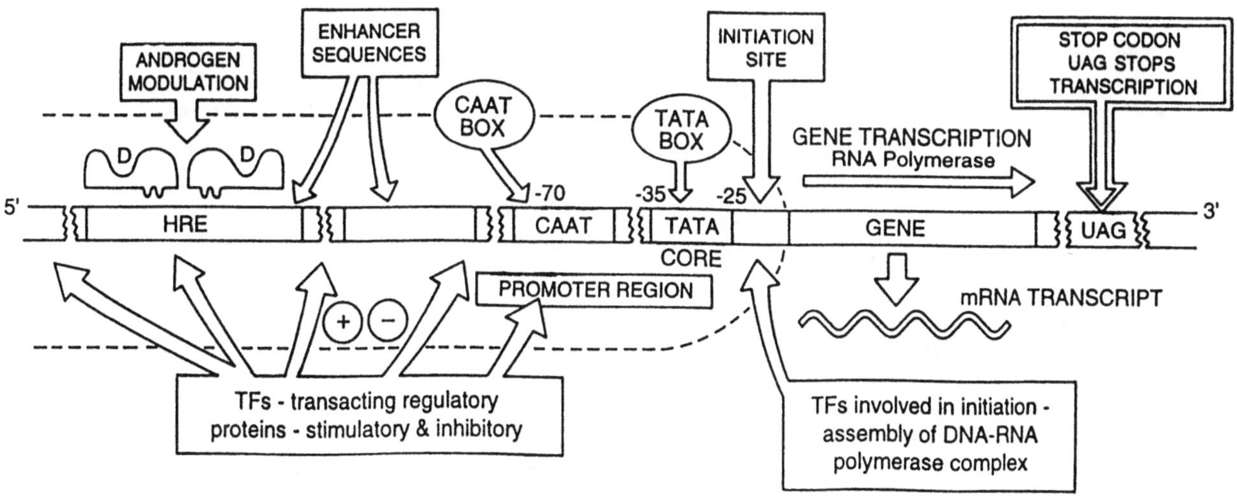

Fig. 6. Diagrammatic representation of the promoter region of a gene showing various cis-acting enhancer sequences, and indicating that various stimulatory and inhibitory, trans-acting growth factors can influence gene transcription

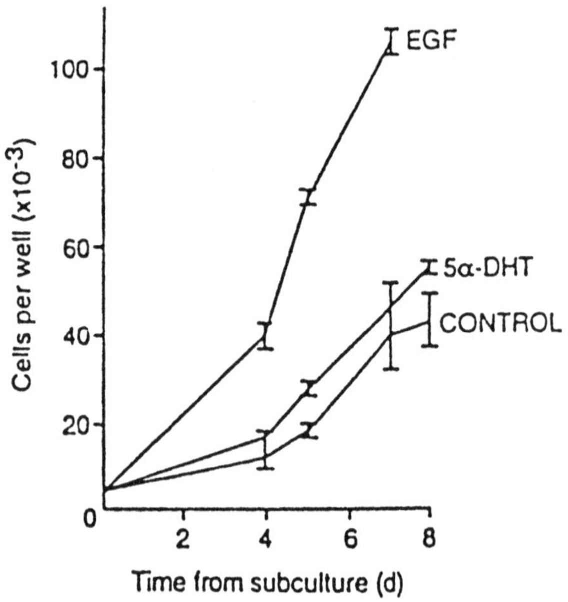

Fig. 7. Various growth factors stimulate cell proliferation of normal prostatic epithelial cells (CAPE cell line) in culture, whereas DHT has little, if any, effect

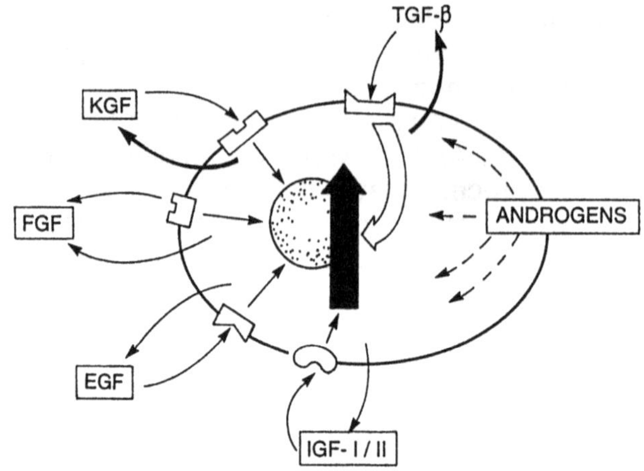

Fig. 8. Prostatic growth relates to a balance between the mitogenic effects of certain growth factors against the restraint exercised by others, under the modulating influence of androgens

The multifocal origin of prostate cancer is of interest and the propensity for cancer to develop in the transition and peripheral zones of the gland requires consideration. It is reasonable to assume that cancer will develop in areas of actively proliferating epithelial cells, regions of hyperplasia in which "genetic aberrations" would occur, with epithelial cell proliferation a consequence of a dysfunctional imbalance in the normal growth regulatory processes of the prostate.

DHT would therefore seem to be intimately involved in the initiation and early phases of BPH and prostatic cancer pathogenesis although, paradoxically, there is now considerable evidence that normal prostatic cells in culture do not directly respond to androgens, but that cell proliferation is observed only in response to various growth factors (Fig. 7) [39, 46]. Growth regulatory factors which may either stimulate or restrain cell proliferation [47-49] are involved in normal cellular processes, but clearly must also be involved in the pathogenesis of BPH and prostatic cancer. Various peptides have been isolated from the prostate [47] and specific receptors for some of these factors have been identified on cell membranes: some peptides appear to be secreted from the gland. Current research [39,46] directs attention to the growth stimulatory activity of certain of these peptides (Fig. 8), such as epidermal growth factor (EGF), the insulin-like growth factors (IGF) I and II and keratinocyte growth factor (KGF): all are mitogenic in cultures of normal prostate epithelial cells. The capacity of transforming growth factor-ß (TGF-ß) to inhibit epithelial cell proliferation is also well recognised [50,51] and information is rapidly accumulating on the roles of these various regulatory peptides in the complex inter- and intracellular signalling processes of the gland.

An important aspect of growth regulation in the prostate concerns the interactive relationship between the epithelial and stromal compartments of the gland [52]. The innovative, elegant studies of Cunha highlighted a dependency, originally described by Franks [53], of epithelial growth on stromal tissue. It would now seem that androgen-dependent mediators of stromal origin influence biological processes in the epithelium; these mediators are growth stimulatory factors, produced by the stroma, that regulate epithelial proliferation (Fig. 9). Although such studies were directed to the embryonic development of the prostate gland, and indicated that these inductive signalling pathways were important determinants of growth and differentiation, it now seems reasonable to conclude that this interrelationship between stromal and epithelial elements forms part of the normal adult growth regulatory mechanism of the prostate [39]. In a similar manner, oestrogen receptors localised primarily in the stromal compartment [54] could elicit a

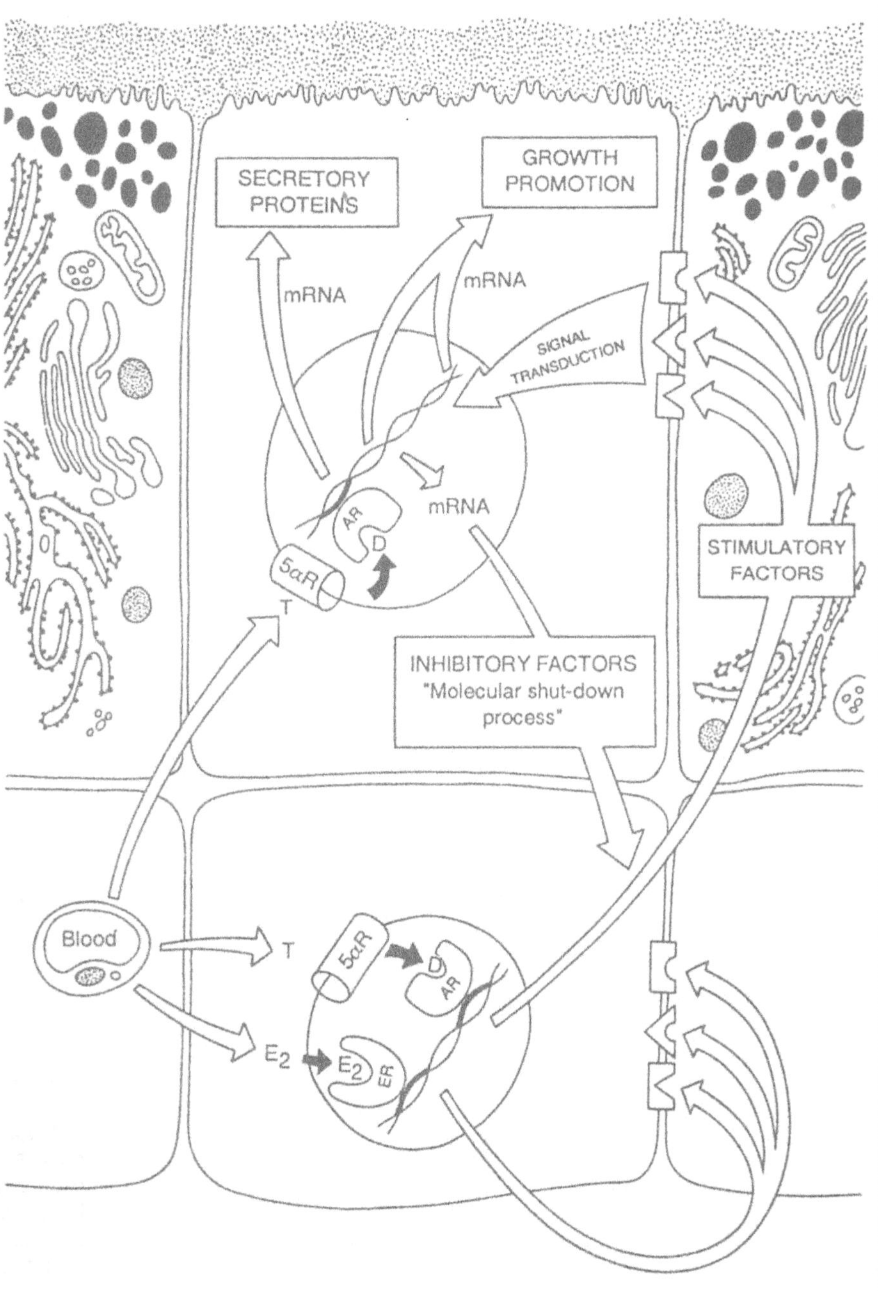

Fig. 9. A simple illustration indicating that androgen-dependent mediators of stromal origin influence epithelial proliferation and prostate growth. It is reasonable to presume that the system encodes for a "molecular shut-down" process, once normal size is attained and homeostasis is established. Receptors for oestrogens are seen localised in the stromal elements, whereas those for DHT are found in both stromal and epithelial compartments

paracrine "oestrogenic effect" on the epithelium by the production of stimulatory or inhibitory factors, or alternately, exercise an autocrine influence on the growth of the stromal elements (Fig. 9).

Although these growth stimulatory factors must be involved in the rapid growth phase of the prostate from adolescence to the early 20s, as epithelium-lined ducts are laid down in a bed of stroma, the precise roles of the various peptides remain to be defined. The intraglandular concentration of EGF is reduced by castration of the male rat [55], with a concomitant increase in available EGF-receptor (EGF-R) concentration [56]. Levels of EGF in prostatic fluid are high [57] and EGF-R has been identified in prostatic epithelium [58,59], possibly confined to basal cells or the basement membrane region of glandular epithelial cells [58], but absent in stromal elements.

It has been established [60] that conditioned media from fibroblasts in culture exercised a mitogenic effect on isolated prostatic epithelial cells in culture. Studies of the Tenovus labora-

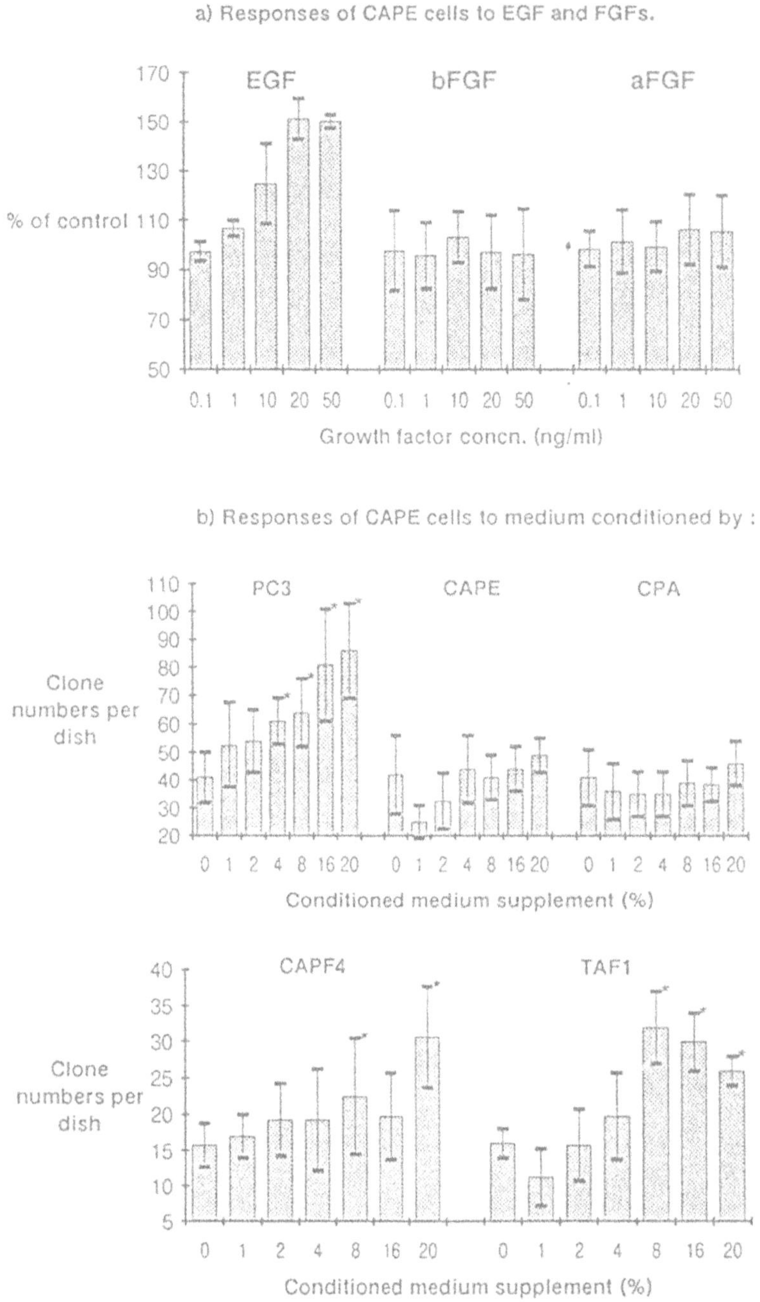

Fig. 10. Normal prostatic epithelial cells (CAPE cell line) respond in culture to EGF but not FGF. Conditioned medium from cultures with the PC3 cancer cell line promotes growth, as does medium from fibroblast cultures (CAPF4 & TAF1), but not that from cultures of CAPE cells, nor from the CPA cancer cell line

tories illustrate this effect (Fig. 10) using normal prostate epithelial cells in culture [61]. The lack of an effect of acidic FGF (FGF-1) or basic FGF (FGF-2) on epithelial cell proliferation is interesting in relation to recent studies which have focussed on KGF, a member of the FGF family, and referred to as FGF-7, which does promote normal epithelial proliferation [62]. KGF is produced by prostatic fibroblasts in culture, where its expression appears to be regulated by androgens. The growth stimulatory effect of KGF on epithelial cells in culture is also inhibited by TGF-ß. KGF is not mitogenic for stromal cells. The IGFs are also potential mitogens in prostatic epithelium [63] although the origin of their synthesis and secretion and bioavailability in the gland remains to be determined [39,64]. Prostatic fibroblasts have been recently shown to produce IGF-II in cell culture, a peptide considered to be involved in the fetal development of the urogenital sinus [65,66]. The inappropriate expression of IGF-II may reflect a more fetal type of phenotype in which new glandular tissue is being generated, but it is noteworthy that seminal plasma contains IGF-I and II, together with the IGF-binding proteins (IGF-BP2, BP3 and BP4), the latter also produced by prostate cells [67]. The IGF-BPs exercise a potentially inhibitory influence, regulating the amount of bioavailable IGF for interaction with cell membrane receptors. The concept that PSA acts as an IGF-BP protease to modify the binding avidity of the IGF-BP for the IGFs, thereby influencing the inhibitory capacity of the IGF-BPs, is interesting [68].

Once the adult prostate size is attained in the early 20s, it must be assumed that homeostasis is then established with a downregulation of growth stimulatory processes. A balance would be established between cell proliferation and programmed cell death, reflected in a balance between growth stimulatory and growth inhibitory factors. The biologically TGF-ß family clearly assumes an important role in the regulation of prostate growth. TGF-ß generally restrains epithelial growth [50,51], is involved in the process of programmed cell death and may well be involved in the "molecular stop mechanism" (Fig. 9) as normal size is attained and homeostasis is established.

Potential for Imbalance in Growth Regulatory Systems

Microscopic BPH, recognised in the early 20s and increasing in prevalence with age [31], must be a consequence of a cellular imbalance whereby proliferative factors override those concerned with growth restraint, suggesting that homeostasis is not always readily established or effectively sustained. Impairment of such multicomponent intercellular signalling processes could readily provoke a proliferative response, with the promotion of epithelial hyperplasia. Noteworthy, for example, are studies [69] in which the int-2 proto-oncogene was introduced into transgenic mice. The enhanced expression of this gene, which encodes for FGF-3, resulted in epithelial hyperplasia. Moreover, FGF has been shown to be mitogenic in certain prostatic cancer cells [70].

Of particular interest, however, has been the characterisation [71] of KGF (FGF-7), which is expressed by rat stromal cells in an androgen-sensitive manner and which stimulates epithelial but not stromal proliferation [62]. Moreover, prostate epithelial cells express a splice variant of one of the four FGF receptor (FGF-R) genes, the FGF-R2(bek) gene, which specifically recognises KGF [72]. Both FGF-1 [73] and FGF-2 [74] are mitogenic for prostate stromal cells. Alternate splicing results in the possibility of four distinct FGF-R genes being expressed, which exhibit structural heterogeneity in the extracellular FGF-binding domain and in the intracellular signal transduction domain [75,76]. Studies on liver cells [77,78] indicate that the different receptor phenotypes can elicit either a stimulatory or inhibitory signal in response to the different FGFs, and it is interesting that, whereas the KGF-specific FGF-R2-exonIIIb is expressed in the slow growing, non-metastatic, well differentiated Dunning R-3327PAP prostate tumour, it is not present in the fast growing undifferentiated cancer. In this metastatic cancer, the expression of the FGF-R2exonIIIc was recognised, a receptor with high binding affinity for bFGF (FGF-2). These tumours also express the FGF-R1(flg) gene encoding a receptor normally recognised in stromal cells [79,80].

Such complex receptors derived from genes with multiple exons (Fig. 11) can therefore lead to structural variation and ligand specificity for the FGF family members as a result of differential splicing of transcripts. It is interesting to speculate on the biological effects of these multiple autocrine or intracrine loops, which result in alterations in the FGF-R family; these alterations might underlie early imbalance of the normal growth regulatory processes of the prostate, leading to epithelial hyperplasia and ultimately to malignancy and androgen-insensitive autonomy of clones of tumour cells. An early report from these laboratories referring to an increased specific binding capacity of tissue preparations from grade II and III prostatic cancers for radiolabelled IGF-I relative to that found for tissue samples from grade I cancer or for BPH samples, simply indicates that imbalance in growth control may involve many components [63].

Possible Cellular Origins of Prostatic Cancer

The fine-tuning of the growth regulatory processes established at homeostasis would be sustained by the balance between stimulatory and inhibitory factors, cellular components that

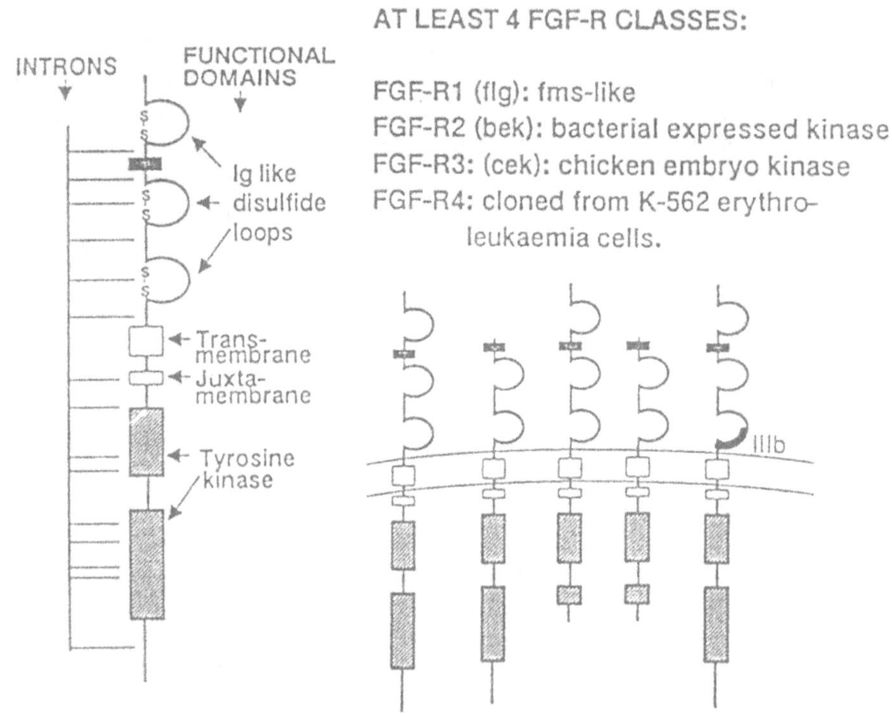

Fig. 11. Diagrammatic illustration of the complexity of the structures of the various FGF receptors, showing external domains that bind FGF and heparin, the trans- and juxta-membrane domains and the intracellular tyrosine kinase. The different splice variants would elicit different ligand specificities

influence cell proliferation or programmed cell death [50]. The dysregulation of intracellular signalling processes leading to epithelial hyperplasia could relate to either an enhanced stimulatory influence or a relative inefficacy of growth restraining factors, the proliferative factors overriding growth restraint leading to microscopic BPH. It seems reasonable to conclude that the origins of the transition zone cancers could well be associated with these areas of hyperplasia in the prostates of younger men.

The well established age-related risk factor associated with the aetiology of clinical BPH would appear to involve the midlife change in the oestrogen-androgen balance, resulting in an enhanced oestrogenic status in later life that promotes a stromally-biased oestrogenic effect [39,46], a consequence of the localisation of oestrogen receptor in the stromal elements (Fig. 9) [54]. Currently available evidence directs attention to the possible synergistic effects of androgen and oestrogen that may be implicated in the development of the prostatic adenoma, more often composed of predominantly stromal tissue and often associated with bladder outflow obstruction [46]. Whether oestradiol promotes the synthesis and secretion of FGF, accepted as a potential autocrine mediator of stromal growth [81], is still to be determined. FGF production by fibroblasts has been reported to be regulated by TGF-ß [82]. The concept, therefore, is not that clinical BPH is causally related to cancer, but the early foci of epithelial hyperplasia are the potential lesions in which cancer might be initiated.

Noteworthy in relation to growth regulation in the prostate are studies directing attention to the regional variation within the rat ductal system of the gland [83-85]. It is reported that active epithelial proliferation is recognised in the distal tip, programmed cell death in the proximal region, nearest the urethra, whereas the major proportion of the ductal epithelial cells, those in the intermediate segment, are maintained in a differentiated state undergoing active secretion. Different patterns of cellular behaviour are therefore observed, with cells presumably receiving the same level of androgenic support. Locally regulated cell-cell interaction with particular regional stromal-epithelial relationships and varying cell-specific responsiveness to androgen modulation must therefore pertain. The active epithelial cell proliferation in the distal tip of the duct may be relevant in relation to the propensity of the peripheral zone to develop cancer.

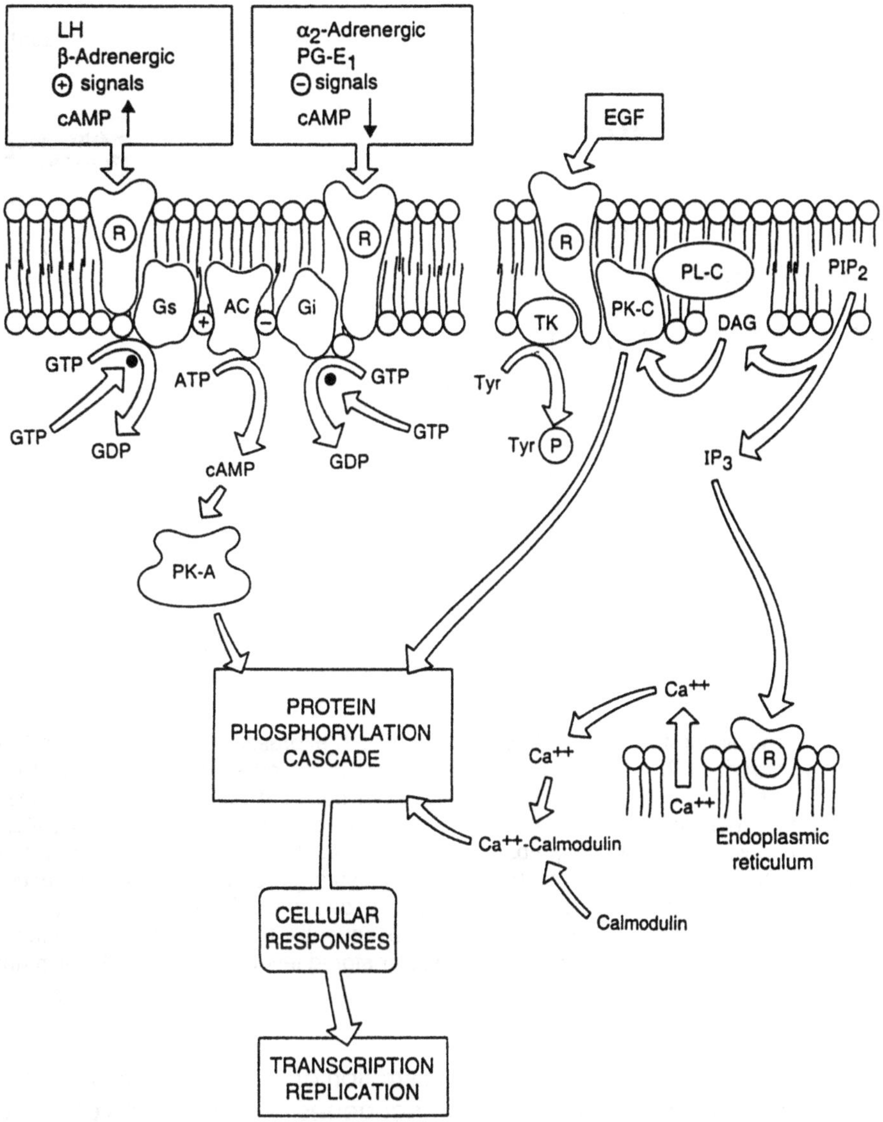

Fig. 12. Representation of complex intracellular signal induction pathways

Growth Regulatory Pathways

Membrane-associated receptors for many growth regulatory factors have been identified in prostatic tissue [47]. The mitogenic signals initiated by the binding of growth factor to the external domain of the receptor (Fig. 12) are transmitted through the intracellular signal transduction pathways to the nucleus, where proto-oncogene activation and gene transcription occurs [86]. It is now realised [87,88] that the oncogenes of the acutely transforming retroviruses are transduced cognates of normal cellular genes, proto-oncogenes like c-*myc*, c-*fos* and c-*jun*, which are intrinsically involved in the regulatory processes concerned with growth and differentiation. These normal cellular homologues encode growth regulatory factors, growth factor receptors, components of the signal transduction pathways, as well as various transcription factors. A better understanding of these intracellular relationships is now providing a greater insight into the consequences of their impairment in disease processes. Such impairment of proto-oncogene function, through point mutations, deletions or amplification, affecting the structure or expression of normal growth regulatory genes, gives rise to the oncogenes, which are then implicated in carcinogenesis. Subversion of growth regulatory processes therefore leads to malignancy.

The nuclear proto-oncogenes c-*myc*, c-*fos* and c-*jun* encode proteins involved in the regulation of gene transcription. They represent some of the earliest genes to be expressed in the

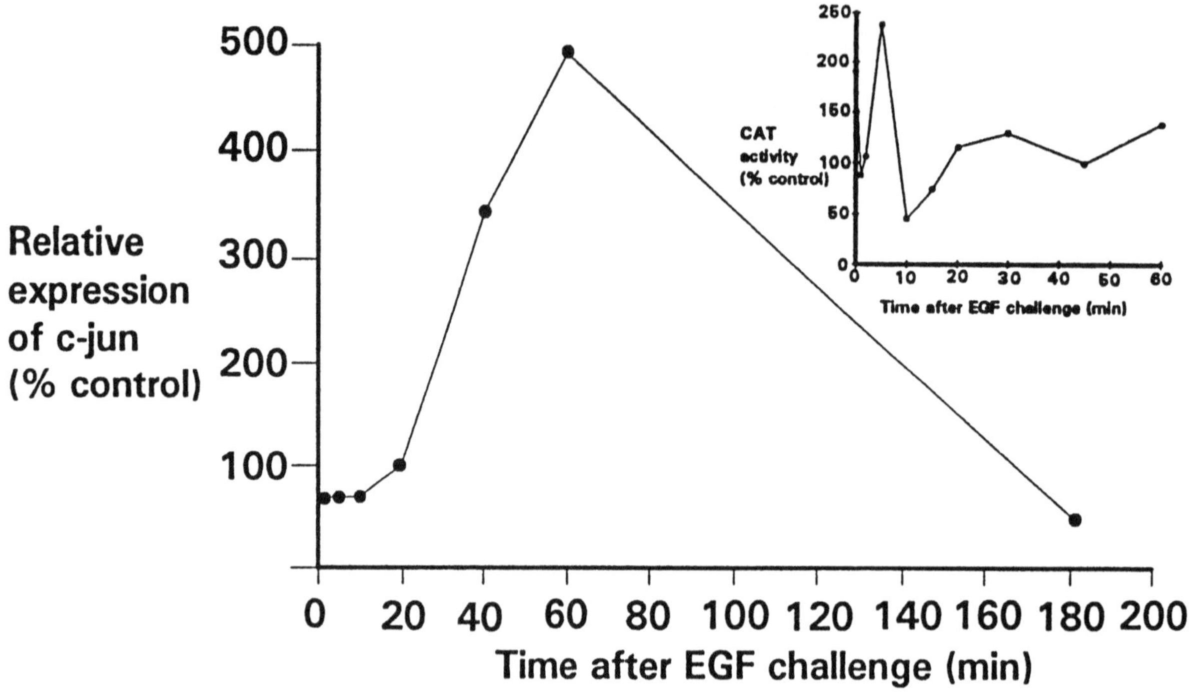

Fig. 13. This illustrates the induction of c-*jun* mRNA expression (main graph) and the activity of a transfected reporter gene construct (TRE-CAT) which was designed to be potentially modulated by *fos/jun* product complexes when experimentally introduced into living cells. Both series of experiments from the Tenovus laboratories used non-neoplastic prostatic epithelial cells (CAPE cell line) challenged with EGF in culture. Upregulation of c-*jun* transcript levels, relative to controls, was observed between 40 and 60 minutes post-treatment. Increases in the activity of the potential *fos/jun* protein product, observed by measuring reporter gene activity, occurred 5 minutes post-treatment. The data suggest that there are significant levels of *fos/jun* products in the cells, prior to challenge, that can be rapidly activated in response to the EGF stimulus. Subsequently, the transcription of at least one *fos/jun* family member, c-*jun*, is elevated, presumably to replenish intracellular stored levels of c-*jun* products in order to sustain the capacity for rapid response to EGF

prostate of castrated rats after administration of androgens [89,90]. These proto-oncogenes transduce the extranuclear mitogenic signals (Fig. 13) into the expression of genes which then encode the transcription factors, the *fos*, *jun* and *myc* proteins which regulate the expression of secondary genes concerned with growth. The *fos* and *jun* proteins are the principal components of the AP-1 transcription factor (Fig. 14). The *jun* protein binds to the activating protein (AP-1) response elements (AP-1RE) as a homodimer, whereas the *fos* protein associates with *jun* as a heterodimer in order to modulate gene activity [91,92]. The protein-protein association is a particular specific interaction of the "leucine zipper" structural domains of the two proteins [93]. Other proteins such as the steroid receptors can modulate, possibly inhibit, the *jun*-promoted transcription by way of a similar protein-protein or *jun*-receptor interaction on the DNA enhancer sequences (Fig. 13). It is envisaged that c-*fos* and c-*jun* play a pivotal role in these complex prostatic regulatory systems, with the *fos* and *jun* proteins being recruited to interact with AR in adjacent flanking positions on the AREs (Fig. 15) [94].

EGF and FGF induce c-*fos* and c-*jun* genes, stimulatory effects leading to cellular proliferation unless the inhibitory influence of factors such as TGF-ß prevails. In this finely-tuned, complex regulatory process, the *fos* and *jun* proteins autoregulate the expression of their own genes (Fig. 14).

Other growth restraining proteins relate to the so-called "tumour suppressor genes" such as *p53* and the retinoblastoma (*Rb*) genes. Somatic cell hybridisation studies [95] focussed on the fusion of normal cells with tumour cells, produced hybrid cells with restricted tumorigenicity. These studies provided evidence of such growth restraining genes, now recognised

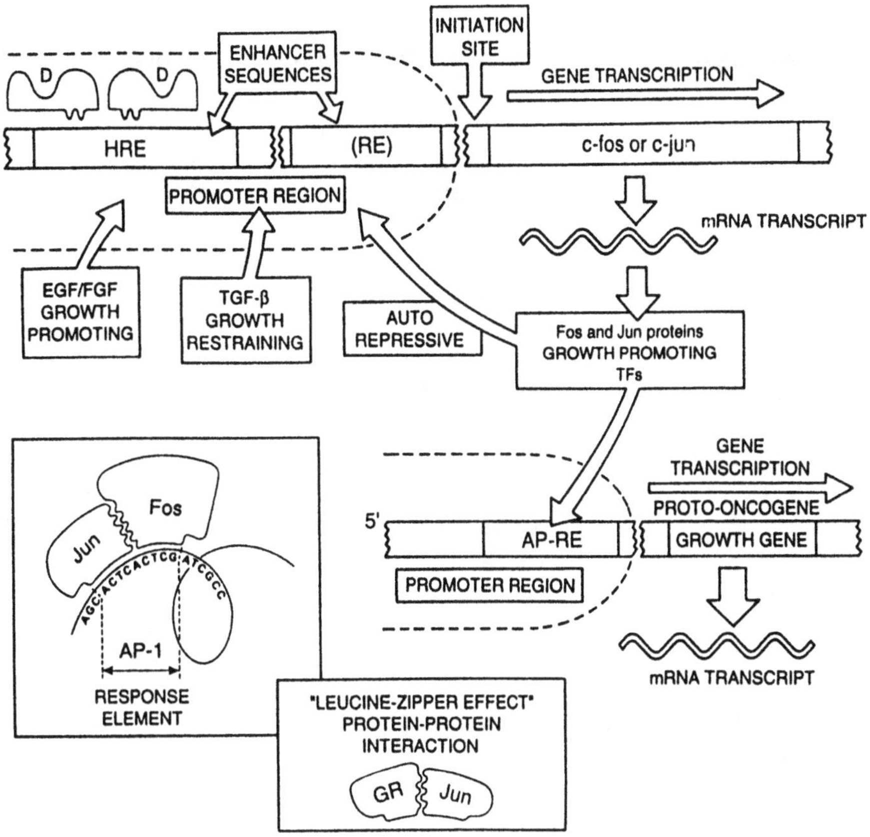

Fig. 14. The androgen-modulated expression of a c-*fos* or c-*jun* gene, encoding for proteins which autoregulate the expression of their own gene and influence the transcriptional activity of other genes concerned with growth regulation. The concept of leucine-zipper interactions and *fos-jun* dimers is diagrammatically illustrated

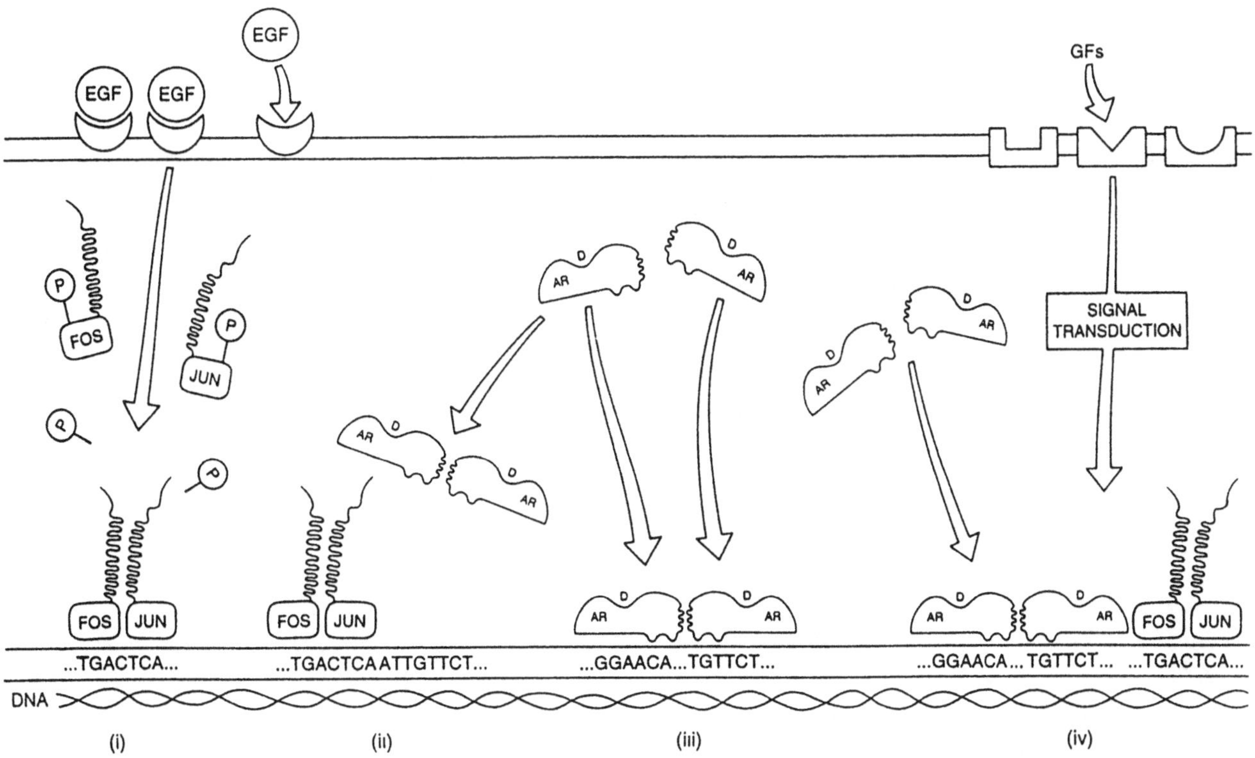

Fig. 15. Growth factors (GFs) such as EGF bind to receptors on the cell surface, with greater binding affinity obtained by receptor aggregation. Signal transduction results in the activation of genes like c-*fos* and c-*jun*, which, as heterodimers, bind the AP-1 response elements, characterised by the TGACTCA motif (i). The DHT-AR dimers associate with the AREs characterised by the 15-base pair sequence of GGAACA NNN TGTTCT (iii), two 6-bp half sites separated by a 3-bp spacer. The DHT-ARs may cooperate with the *fos* and *jun* proteins to stimulate gene transcription (iv), or it may be that transcription factors compete for the response elements (ii)

as an integral part of the normal growth regulatory processes. Loss of these genes by mutation or deletion will thereby remove the growth restraining influence on proliferation. A mutant protein expressed as a result of an exon deletion of the *Rb* gene has been reported in the DU145 prostatic cell line [96]. Moreover, transfection of the cloned normal *Rb* gene into the tumour cells in nude mice suppressed tumorigenicity. There is evidence that the *Rb* protein may modulate c-*myc* expression, either directly or possibly by association with the c-*myc* encoded protein, such that the levels of *myc* protein are controlled [28]. Deletion of the *Rb* gene and loss of the suppressor protein would consequently lead to *myc* activation and enhanced cell proliferation. Alternatively, deletion of a negative *cis*-acting regulator sequence upstream of c-*myc*, through which a trans-acting inhibitor such as TGF-ß restrains gene expression, could equally induce *myc* activity. Allelic deletions on chromosome 13, the location of the *Rb* gene, have been reported [97].

Early Prostate Cancer: Potential for Treatment

There is still a great deal to be learned about the natural history of prostatic cancer (Fig. 16). Androgen ablative therapy effectively produces symptomatic relief in a majority of patients with advanced prostatic cancer, although the disease quickly progresses, presumably as clones of androgen-unresponsive cells develop. Clearly, however, a large proportion of the cancer cells at this stage of the disease do respond to the withdrawal of androgen. Continual discussion centres on the clinical value of "complete androgen blockade" [30,98] by means of an LHRH analogue in association with an antiandrogen, and it would appear that there is a group of patients, possibly those with the more differentiated, androgen-responsive cancer, who do benefit from this form of treatment. Current interest also centres on the recognition of confined cancer by early screening initiatives [99,100], with radical prostatectomy [101] or radiotherapy [102] as treatment options. Controversy would be evoked by the concept that endocrine therapy in the form of, for example, a 5α-reductase inhibitor together with low-dose antiandrogen, might offer an equally acceptable and effective form of treatment. Despite early recognition, the disease is often not confined but has disseminated prior to therapy and this form of androgen blockade, once evaluated, could offer complete androgen deprivation while maintaining normal levels of testosterone in plasma [103].

It is not unreasonable to investigate the potential benefits of the 5α-reductase inhibitor-antiandrogen combination as adjuvant therapy following radical prostatectomy for confined cancer. Where dissemination has occurred, the effect of early endocrine treatment on foci of

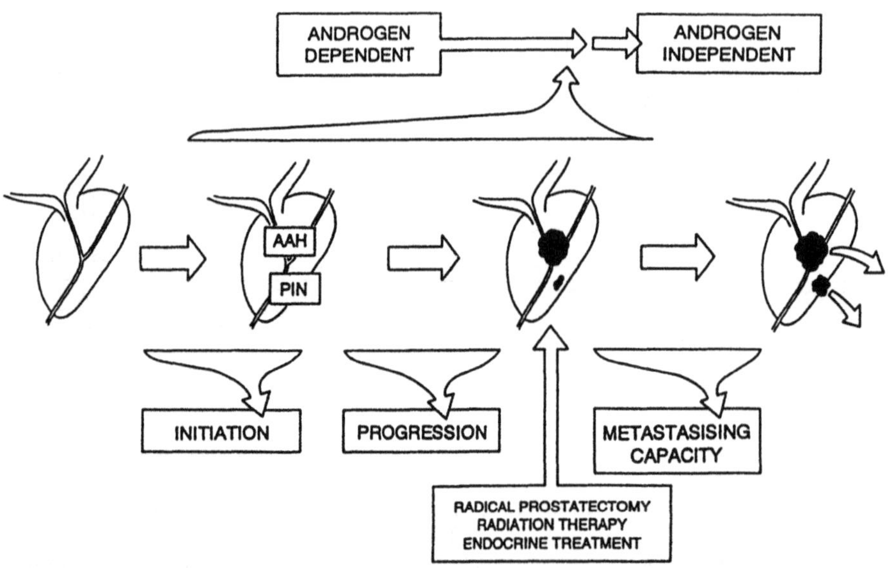

Fig. 16. The natural history of prostatic cancer

metastatic, possibly androgen-sensitive cells could be beneficial and the results of preliminary studies suggest that this approach is effective [104]. A secondary issue relates to the potential of the combination regimen as intervention therapy for the more aggressive AAH and PIN lesions. It is important to determine the influence of early androgen withdrawal on the subsequent behaviour of latent carcinoma. Of paramount importance, however, with such exciting treatment options is that the fundamental biochemical and endocrine processes involved in the hormonal regulation of prostatic growth and function are better understood. The complexity and sophistication of these physiological interactions that modulate cellular behaviour are well recognised [105], as is the potential for new, more rational forms of therapy as growth dysregulation is understood.

In recognising that carcinogenesis is a complex multi-step process from initiation, through promotion and progression to the invasive metastatic disease, it is clear that the focus of attention must be on the initial molecular changes. Although accepting that prostatic cancer can only be cured if confined to the gland [30,98], it is this search for early cancer which will be invaluable in the provision of tissue to support investigations into the molecular basis of the disease.

Prostate Growth Regulation: Fine-Tuning by Androgens

The past decade has seen the isolation and characterisation of growth regulatory factors and their receptors in prostate tissue [47], the cloning of steroid receptor genes [106] and the identification of oncogenes and some tumour suppressor genes, an exponential increase in knowledge [107-109], but interest now centres on understanding their function and interrelationships, particularly within the prostate gland. As stated, however, the essential feature of the prostate is its dependence on a continual presentation of androgens to maintain structure and function, although the adult gland is sustained within a multihormonal environment, with the capacity to respond to a wide range of growth factors. It would seem that the specificity of the hormonal response in the various cells of the gland depends on the accessibility of genomic sequences and the array of growth factors available to the cells. Androgens are necessary for proliferation, but proliferation is not an inevitable consequence of the presence of androgen, nor of the DHT-AR complex, and it is clear that other determinant factors are involved. The androgenic influence exercised by DHT on cellular responses depends on the specific recognition by DHT-AR (Fig. 4) of the DNA nucleotide sequences referred to as HREs [42-45], or more specifically in the prostate, as AREs.

Gene specificity relates to the various DNA regulatory enhancer sequences in the promoter region [110] and their linear disposition or spatial arrangement (Figs. 7 and 20). There is a marked homology [111] between the nucleotide sequences (GREs) that associate with the receptors for glucocorticoids (GR), androgens (AR) and progesterone (PR), whereas the oestrogen receptor (ER) recognises another distinct sequence of nucleotides (ERE). Other factors certainly play a rôle in determining the specificity of the cell's response to steroid hormones; for example, some studies show that despite the presence in a gene promoter region of both GREs and EREs, activation was only seen with oestrogens [112]

The structure of the AR protein deduced from the sequences of the cloned AR cDNA from rat [113,114] and human [115-117] prostate tissue conforms with the functional modularity described for other steroid receptors (Fig. 17) [106]. The human AR is a 110 kDa protein encoded by a single copy gene located on the X chromosome and extending over more than 90kb [116-119]. The coding sequence is divided into 8 exons with introns positioned in a manner similar to other steroid receptor genes [119-121]. The sequence encoding the N-terminal region comprises one large exon [122], the two DNA binding zinc fingers are encoded separately by two small exons, and the information for the DHT binding domain is separated into 4 exons [119,122-124].

The functional domains of the AR exercise a major controlling influence on the association with the HREs. The DHT binding domain is located at the carboxy-terminal region (Fig. 17). Association with DHT triggers the transcription activation function of the AR, reveals dimerisation domains or interfaces, and the conformational change unmasks the DNA binding domain of the receptor which is characterised by

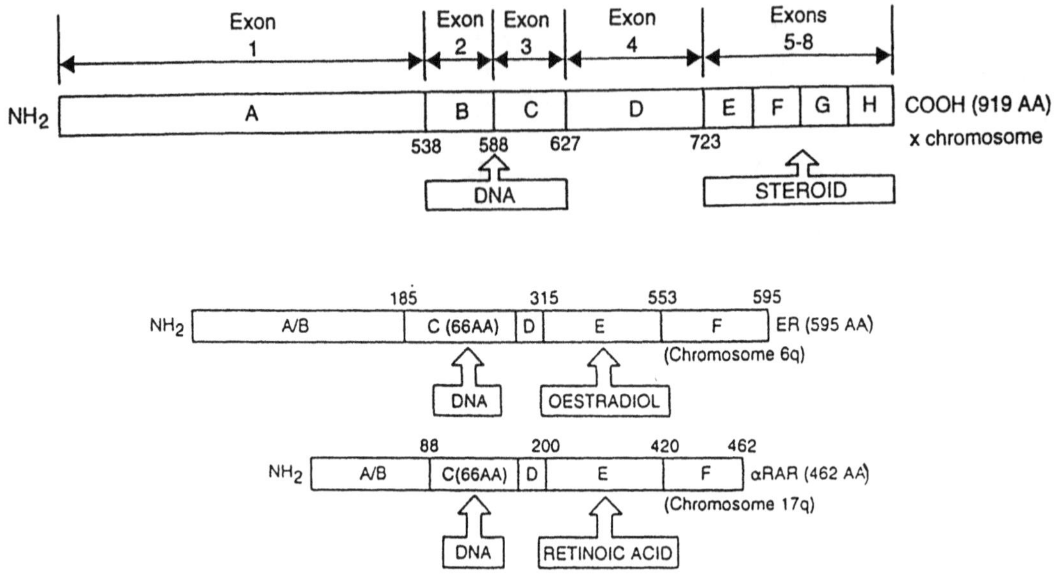

Fig. 17. Simple schematic representation of the structure of the androgen receptor relative to the size of certain other human nuclear receptors

the pair of zinc fingers [123]. As with other transcription factors, the DHT-AR contains sequences of amino acids rich in cysteine residues, 4 in the N-terminal (CI) zinc finger and 5 in the second (CII) C-terminal finger. The coordinate binding between cysteines and zinc forms the zinc fingers, which loop into major grooves of the DNA double helix (Fig. 18) where they specifically recognise individual base pairs.

The AR, without DHT bound, is in an inactive conformational state, associated with hsp90 [33-36]. A region of the GR believed to associate with hsp90 has been mapped to the C-terminal region [125]. After DHT binding, the hsp90 dissociates (Fig. 4) and an AR homodimer is formed, the structure of which is stabilised by association with AREs [126]. One dimerisation interface is sited in the DNA binding domain between cysteines 1 and 2 in the CII zinc finger [127]. The second, probably more important interface, overlaps with the steroid binding domain and is DHT inducible [128].

The particular dyad symmetry of the HREs (Figs. 15 and 20) relates to the binding of DHT-AR as a dimer, the dimer structure conferring stability to the transcription complex of RNA polymerase, DNA and the various associated transcription factors including the steroid receptors. The principal DHT-inducible transcription activation function of the AR is localised to the steroid binding domain, with a second in the N-terminal region considered to constitutively confer promoter-selective, trans-acting transcription

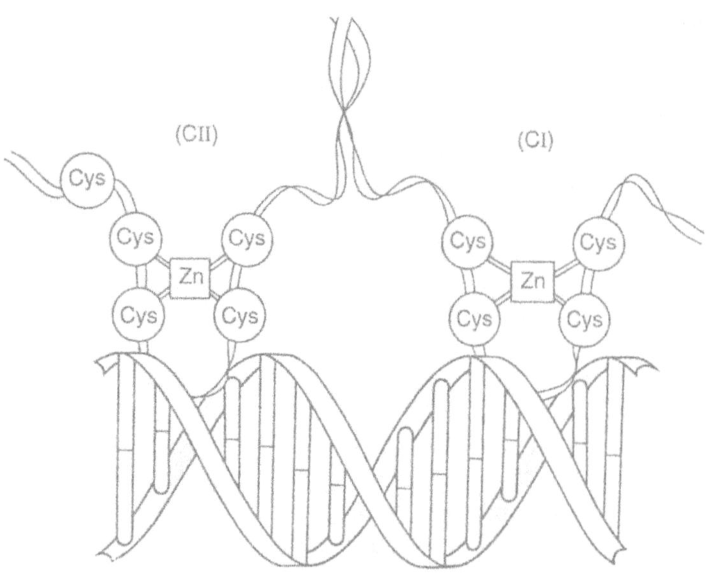

Fig. 18. Schematic concept of the "zinc fingers" fitting into the major grooves of DNA

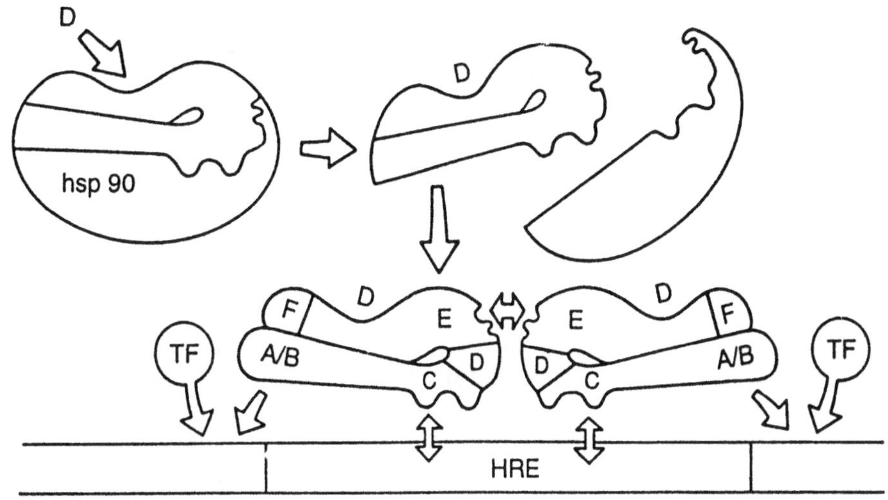

Fig. 19. Diagrammatic concept of the association between DHT-AR dimers and AREs, illustrating dimerisation interfaces, and a transcription activation function relating to the N-terminal region. The F segment represents the F, G and H regions

activation [129-132]. Some of the interrelationships are diagrammatically illustrated in Figure 15 and Figure 19, which simply indicate the influence of DHT-AR association with AREs in recruiting other transcription factors to the promoter region.

The HREs for GR and ER were some of the first to be studied [37,42,132,133] and since the HREs for GR, PR and AR are highly homologous [111], it was not surprising that AR appeared to function through the GREs of the tyrosine aminotransferase (TAT) gene [134] and the mouse mammary tumour virus (MMTV) long-term repeat (LTR) region [135-137].

The putative AREs in the prostate binding protein (PBP) gene [138] resemble in structure, at least with regard to the TGTTCT motif (Figs.14 and 19) at the right hand of the 15-bp consensus sequence [111,139], the HREs of the TAT and MMTV LTR promoter regions. The spatial orientation of the AR homodimer supports the association with the two 6-bp half-sites separated by a 3-bp spacer [37]. One half of the dimer recognises the specific half-site sequence, the other binding less effectively to the imprecise half, cooperative binding being probably assisted by protein-protein interactions within the dimer. Some HREs exist only as half-palindromes [140] and in the MMTV LTR promoter region (Fig. 20) there are four HREs, with HRE3 and HRE4 being 6-bp half-sites. A gradation of response to androgens has been reported through the four HREs of the promoter [136] and a possible requirement for the spatial juxtaposition of the DNA response elements to exercise an optimal effect [111] is suggested by the disposition of multiple HREs [133,141,142]. The co-existence of AREs alongside clusters of transcription factor binding sites suggests functional synergism

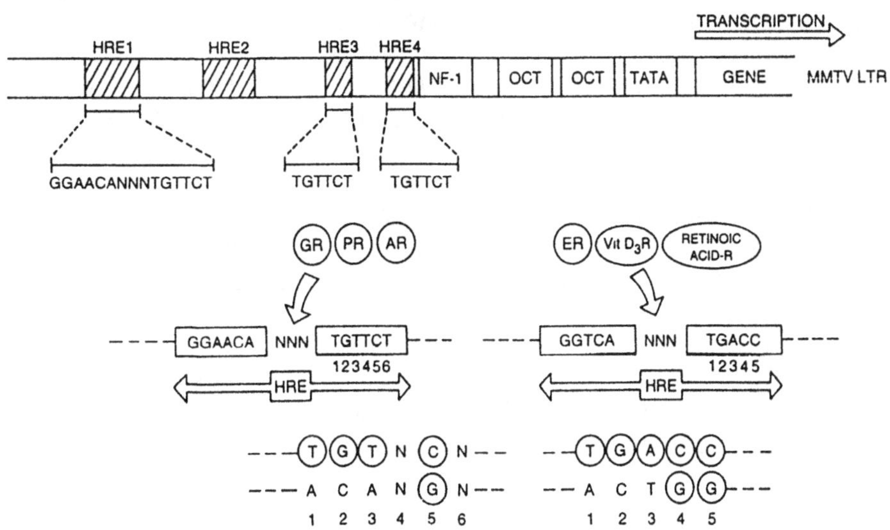

Fig. 20. The promoter region of the MMTC LTR gene showing enhancer sequences and HRE half-sites. The HREs for different receptors are illustrated, together with a simple representation of the important bases of the HREs which make contact with the receptor amino acids

[110,143,144], and results from the Tenovus laboratories [47] show that the binding of AR to HREs is favoured in the presence of NF-1 and NF-3 consensus sequences. Association of NF-1 transcription factor [145] or the ER [146] with enhancer sequences changes their spatial orientation or "bends" the DNA.

Since the GREs and EREs differ in only a few nucleotides [147], it would appear that just as the receptor gene superfamily has evolved [106], so too probably has a family of nucleotide sequences diverged to ensure tissue and gene specificity in the response to steroid hormones.

The consensus sequence GGAACA NNN TGTTCT responds to GR, PR and AR, whereas GGTCA NNN TGACC recognises ER as well as receptors for vitamin D3, retinoic acid and thyroid hormones (Fig. 20), the important differences being at nucleotides 3 and 4 of the right hand half-site. Mutation analysis and DNA binding and gene transfer studies [43,148,149] established that symmetrical HREs containing an adenine (A) residue at the nucleotide 3 position, bound ER but not PR [147,150], whereas a thymine (T) residue at 3 was necessary for PR binding. The nucleotide at position 4 can be T or cytosine (C) in GREs, AREs or PREs, but must be C in EREs. All receptors contact the 5-methyl group of thymine (T1) in the half-site as well as the N-7 of guanine (G2). The 5-methyl of T3 binds AR, PR and GR but a T3 prevents ER binding [147,150]. The nucleotide at the 4 position is not contacted by PR, AR or PR, but a C4 is essential for ER binding, although it is the opposite strand G4 guanine which is contacted by ER through the N-7 position. A C at the 5 position is important for all HREs, but contact is with the opposite strand G. It would appear that approximately 60% of GREs have T in position 6 of the half-site.

Freedman [151] has recently reviewed his two-dimensional magnetic resonance imaging studies directed to the interaction between HREs and steroid receptors and indicates that particular individual amino acids in the zinc fingers of the DNA binding domain of the receptor protein are specifically implicated in the association. Two amino acid residues between cysteines 3 and 4 of CI zinc finger and the second residue after the fourth cysteine, a valine, have been identified as important, the valine contacting the 5-methyl of the T3 of the GRE half-site (Fig. 20). An alanine residue is reported [152] in the same position of the ER.

Functional Synergism Between Receptors and Transcription Factors

The complexity and sophistication of these steroid hormone modulated gene regulatory processes is now well recognised. Clearly, the androgenic influence on the prostate is dependent on cooperative AREs, associating with DHT-AR, cell-specific transcription factors and optimal spatial orientation of chromatin in the regions associated with the gene promoter that "read" the response signals. The intercession and binding of other growth regulatory transcription factors in juxtapositions flanking the AREs would seem mandatory to the growth regulatory process (Fig. 15) [110]. Such functional synergism would require optimal spatial configuration of the various response elements, although there is evidence of protein-protein (leucine zipper) interaction between receptors and transcription factors, as well as the transcription activation function of the N-terminal region of the AR [130-132], diagrammatically illustrated in Figures 15 and 19.

The association of DHT-AR with AREs therefore induces an effective spatial orientation of the DNA to allow other factors to be recruited to the promoter region. It is yet to be determined whether the association is a transient, intermediary stage in the promotion of gene expression, a process directed primarily to enhancing the accessibility to the genome of the other growth regulatory factors.

Prostate Cancer: Initiation and Progression

The integrated response of cells to signalling language, reading sense from the messages induced by the various growth factors and hormones, is clearly a finely-tuned system. Fundamentally, it malfunctions as proliferative processes override growth restraining influences in epithelial hyperplasia, and as cells escape from growth regulatory control in carcinogenesis. Multistep carcinogenesis relates to a succession of stages in which the activity or structure of particular proto-oncogenes change such that each step induces further changes consistent with cell transformation and the development of the cellular phenotype expressing the full malignant potential. Weinberg [28] refers to cancer as "a complementary misbehaviour" of various oncogenes, an enhanced expression of growth stimulatory genes, and a possible loss of growth suppressor genes. He suggested a two-oncogene concept, whereby two oncogenes acting in concert initiate cancer, genes such as the *ras*-family encoding cytoplasmic proteins [153] homologous with the G-proteins [154] that transduce membrane receptor signals (Fig. 12), and a *myc*-like gene expressing nuclear growth promoting factors [155]. Elevated expression of c-Ha-*ras* is reported in prostate cancer cell lines [156] and the Tenovus laboratories [157] showed that levels of c-Ha-*ras* mRNA transcripts increase with tumour dedifferentiation. Transfection of an activated *ras* oncogene into cancer cell lines increased metastatic potential [158] and in an experimental system, a mouse reconstitution model [159], introduction of *ras* and *myc* together induced actively proliferating prostatic cancer. Elevated *c-myc* mRNA levels have also been demonstrated in prostatic cancer with suggestions [160] that higher concentrations relate to high grade cancer.

Illustrated simply and diagrammatically, Figure 21 suggests that foci of "premalignancy" in areas of hyperplasia may result from genetic instability, with anomalous gene expression such as *ras* activation inducing dysregulation. The activation of *ras* genes in the early phases of carcinogenesis is not sufficient in itself to transform cells [153] and the cooperation of nuclear oncogenes is necessary. Such a premalignant phenotype, even a focus of latent cancer, could also be influenced by the paracrine restraining effects of normal, neighbouring cells, described by Weinberg as "transcending a hostile environment" [28]. Further genetic subversion, possibly activation of nuclear genes, could lead to a more complete overriding of any restraining influences, essentially usurping growth regulatory processes.

Does, therefore, the inappropriate production through exon splicing variation of a less specific FGF receptor in the prostate epithelial cells [62,161,162], a switch from the exclusive expression of exon IIIb to exon IIIc in the FGF-R gene (Fig. 11), constitute one of the earlier molecular events relating to carcinogenesis? Epithelial cells would then be insensitive to stromally-derived KGF (FGF-7). The FGF-R2 (IIIc) splice variant, which recognises bFGF (FGF-2), is implicated in the development of the more aggressive Dunning prostate tumours [161, 162], but are such changes related to epithelial hyperplasia? Does genetic subversion in the form of an aberrant *ras* membrane transducing protein (Fig. 12) induce early premalignant lesions with abnormal triggering of growth factor signals? Does TGF-ß provide a restraining influence on these foci of early cancer, possibly through a regulator sequence on the *myc* gene, or alternately, by the positive control of a secondary gene such as the *Rb* gene that encodes a product that suppresses *myc* activity? Most of these early lesions are slow-growing. Recent studies [163] would also suggest that the putative antimetastatic nm23 protein encoded by the nm23 gene, located on chromosome 17, may also influence the expression of the *myc* gene [164-167].

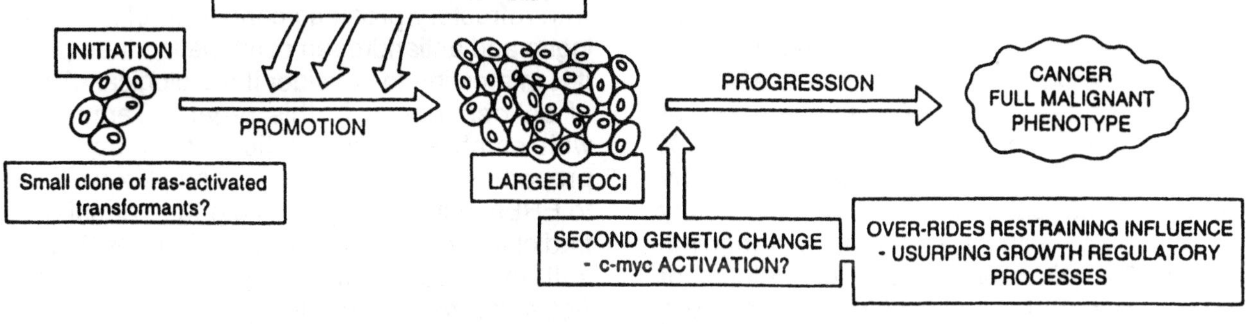

Fig. 21. Simple illustration of possible molecular events that might relate to prostate cancer initiation and promotion

The series of genetic changes involves a transition from relatively slow-growing non-metastatic, androgen-sensitive cancer cells, to a rapidly-growing, androgen-independent malignant tumour. Is the anomalous expression of *myc*, *fos* or *jun*-types of nuclear genes involved in these early phases that lead to the escape from the sophisticated and delicate growth regulatory influence of androgens? These genes clearly play a pivotal role as regulators of proliferation (Figs.13 and 14), promoting the transition of cells from the resting G0 into the G1 state of the cell cycle. Their facultative expression would seem to be under the modulating influence of steroid hormones [168,169] and, as described earlier, their encoded protein products interact with the androgen receptors, as the DHT-ARs recruit transcription factors for the more effective expression of genes concerned with cell proliferation and DNA synthesis. Inappropriate gene expression or gene mutation is associated with constitutive expression, as dependence on androgen decreases and autonomy is realised.
The heterogeneity of advanced metastatic cancer is well accepted [170]. Androgen-dependent cells die in the absence of hormones, whereas the androgen-sensitive cells can survive in the absence of androgens but grow more quickly in their presence. Some cells may be indirectly dependent on androgens, requiring paracrine growth promoting factors from neighbouring androgen-sensitive cells: others may be insensitive to androgens. It is presumed that the autonomous growth of the independent cells results in cancer progression, but do the androgen-sensitive cells adapt to the lower levels of androgen with the constitutive expression of growth-related genes [171]? Can the adaptation of completely androgen-sensitive foci of cancer cells be restrained or prevented by total androgen withdrawal?
Genetic instability of a developing tumour could readily lead to the formation of cell variants with different degrees of sensitivity to androgen, including the production of AR mutants. AR gene deletion has been recognised as one cause of the androgen insensitivity syndrome, an X chromosome-linked disorder characterised by defective masculinisation in karyotypically 46XY subjects with intra-abdominal or inguinal testes [172]. Although the complete deletion of the AR gene and of a complete exon encoding the androgen binding domain of the AR have been reported in relation to the syndrome, most of the mutations are of single base pairs.
Such AR mutants may also be implicated in the changes that cause loss of androgen sensitivity of prostate cancer. A mutant receptor in the LNCaP cancer cell line caused changes in ligand specificity such that growth responses were stimulated by oestrogens, progestins and antiandrogens [173]. PCR single strand conformation polymorphism studies in the Tenovus laboratories [174] on a series of tissue samples from prostate cancers as well as some BPH specimens, recognised in one differentiated cancer a point mutation within the F exon of the steroid binding domain, a C to G at nucleotide 3423. This is predicted to cause an amino acid substitution, glutamine to glutamic acid, at amino acid 798. Band shifts on PCR-SSCP analysis suggest other tumours contain mixtures of mutant and wild-type AR genes. Two of 10 samples of BPH tissue studied contained intronic mutations, one a G to A at position 3746 of intron 6 and the other a C to T at position 2410 of intron 3. Such mutations might introduce alternate splice sites into the AR gene, thereby affecting the structure of the AR protein and mRNA stability. The work confirmed the presence of the previously described LNCaP cell line mutation in the H exon of LNCaP DNA [173].
Moreover, mutant ARs may not be DHT-regulated, but could influence growth regulatory processes by their uncontrolled constitutive activation of androgen responsive genes. Although there is little evidence that the currently available antiandrogens normally elicit agonistic properties [175], their relationship to mutant ARs and the consequent molecular response requires study. The effects of antiandrogens at the molecular level must be defined. Scher [176] has reported clinical responses associated with a decline in serum PSA levels after antiandrogen withdrawal from patients with refractory prostatic cancer on LHRH analogue and antiandrogen combination therapy.
It is interesting to consider the biological effects of antioestrogens in this regard. Tamoxifen, with established agonistic and antagonistic properties [177], binds as a complex with ER to EREs, but does not promote the normal oestradiol-induced conformational changes that result in effective transcriptional activation. Activation relating to the agonistic effect of tamoxifen is through the N-terminal A/B domain

[124] that normally represents 1-10% of the oestradiol-induced response, depending on the particular gene concerned. The new complete antioestrogens such as ICI 164,364 elicit only antagonistic properties and prevent binding of ER to EREs by interfering with receptor dimerisation [178], presumably due to steric hindrance caused by the long 7-alkylamide side-chain attached to the oestradiol molecule [179]. The variable agonistic and antagonistic properties of these antihormones must therefore relate to their influence on the relative N-terminal A/B and steroid binding domain transcription activation functions of receptors, associated with the responses of particular genes and specific cell types. It will be important to exploit this new molecular dimension to our understanding of the mechanisms by which antiandrogens will influence the complex processes of prostatic carcinogenesis.

Acknowledgements

The work concerned with the identification of androgen receptor gene mutations is supported by a Merck, Sharp & Donne Medical School Research Grant. Dr. Bronwen Evans is supported by a grant from the Medical Research Council, United Kingdom, and Dr. C.L. Eaton, Dr. M.E. Harper and Ms Anna Weir by the Tenovus Organisation, Cardiff, Wales.

REFERENCES

1 World Health Organisation: Trends in prostate cancer 1980-1988. WHO Weekly Epidemiological Record 1992 (67):281-288

2 Zaridze DG and Boyle P: Cancer of the prostate: Epidemiology and aetiology. Br J Urol 1987 (59): 493-502

3 Boyle P: The evolution of an epidemic of unknown origin. In: L Denis (ed) Prostate Cancer 2000. European School of Oncology Monographs. Springer-Verlag, New York/Heidlberg/Berlin 1994 pp 5-11

4 Barry MJ, Beckley S, Boyle P et al: Importance of understanding the epidemiology and natural history of BPH. In: Cockett ATK, Aso Y, Chatelain C, Denis L, Griffiths K, Khoury S, Murphy G (eds) Proceedings of the First International Consultation on Benign Prostatic Hyperplasia (BPH), 1991. Publ SCI Paris, Paris 1992 pp 13-21

5 Lytton B, Emery JM, Harvard BM: The incidence of benign prostatic obstruction. J Urol 1968 (99):639-645

6 Glynn RJ, Campion EW, Bouchard GR, Silbert JE: The development of benign prostatic hyperplasia among volunteers in the normative aging study. Am J Epidemiol 1985 (121):78-90

7 Miller JG: Diagnosis of stage A prostate cancer in the people's Republic of China. In: Coffey DS, Resnick MI, Dorr FA, Karr JP (eds) A Multidisciplinary Analysis of Controversies in the Management of Prostatic Cancer. Plenum Press, New York 1988 pp 17-24

8 Haenszel W and Kurihara M: Studies of Japanese migrants. I. Mortality from cancer and other diseases among Japanese in the United States. JNCI 1968 (40):43-68

9 McNeal JE: The zonal anatomy of the prostate. Prostate 1981 (2):35-49

10 Armenian HK, Lilienfeld AM, Diamond EL, Bross IDJ: Relation between benign prostatic hyperplasia and cancer of the prostate: A prospective and retrospective study. Lancet 1974 (ii):115-117

11 Greenwald P, Kirmss V, Polan AK, Dick VS: Cancer of the prostate among men with benign prostatic hyperplasia. JNCI 1974 (53):335-340

12 Bostwick DG, Balcells FS, Cooner WH et al: Benign prostatic hyperplasia (BPH) and cancer of the prostate. In: Cockett ATK, Aso Y, Chatelain C, Denis L, Griffiths K, Khoury S, Murphy G (eds) Proceedings of the First International Consultation on Benign Prostatic Hyperplasia (BPH), 1991. Publ SCI Paris, Paris 1992 pp 139-159

13 McNeal JE, Price HM, Redwine EA, Freiha FS, Stamey TA: Stage A versus stage B adenocarcinoma of the prostate: Morphological comparison and biological significance. J Urol 1988 (139):61-65

14 Kovi J and Mostofi FK: Atypical hyperplasia of prostate. Urology 1989 (34 Suppl):23-27

15 McNeal JE, Bostwick DG, Kindrachuk RA, Redwine EA, Freiha FS, Stamey TA: Patterns of progression in prostate cancer. Lancet 1986 (i):60-63

16 Bostwick DG and Brawer MK: Prostatic intra-epithelial neoplasia and early invasion in prostate cancer. Cancer 1987 (59):788-794

17 McNeal JE and Bostwick DG: Intraductal dysplasia: A premalignant lesion of the prostate. Hum Pathol 1986 (17):54-71

18 Kastendieck H: Correlations between atypical primary hyperplasia and carcinoma of the prostate: A histological study of 180 total prostatectomies. Pathol Res Pract 1980 (169):366-387

19 Baba S: Epidemiology of cancer of the prostate: Analysis of countries of high and low incidence. In: Jacobi GH and Hohenfellner R (eds) Prostate Cancer. International Perspectives in Urology, Vol 3. Williams & Wilkins, Baltimore 1982 pp 11-28

20 Oota K and Misu Y: A study on latent carcinoma of the prostate in Japanese. GANN 1958 (49):283-293

21 Cantrell BB, deKlerk DP, Eggleston JC, Boitnott JK, Walsh PC: Pathological factors that influence prognosis in stage A prostatic cancer: The influence of extent versus grade. J Urol 1981 (125): 516-520

22 Stamey TA: Cancer of the prostate. Monogr Urol 1982 (3):1-10

23 Epstein JI, Paull G, Eggleston JC, Walsh PC: Prognosis of untreated stage A1 prostatic carcinoma: A study of 94 cases with extended followup. J Urol 1986 (136):837-839

24 Whitmore WF Jr: Stage A prostatic cancer (editorial). J Urol 1986 (136):883

25 Huggins C and Hodges CV: Studies on prostatic cancer. I. The effect of castration, of estrogen and of androgen injection on serum phosphatases in metastatic carcinoma of the prostate. Cancer Res 1941 (1):293-297

26 Huggins C, Stevens RE, Hodges CV: Studies on prostatic cancer. Arch Surg 1941 (43):209-223

27 Huggins C: Endocrine-induced regression of cancers. In: Les Prix Nobel, Imprimerie Royale. PA Norstedt & Söner, Stockholm 1967 pp 172-182

28 Weinberg RA: Oncogenes, antioncogenes, and the molecular basis of multistep carcinogenesis. Cancer Res 1989 (49):3713-3721

29 Sager R: Tumor suppressor genes: The puzzle and the promise. Science 1989 (246):1406-1412

30 Denis LJ: Controversies in the management of localised and metastatic prostatic cancer. Eur J Cancer 1991 (27):333-341

31 Isaacs JT and Coffey DS: Etiology and disease process of benign prostatic hyperplasia. Prostate 1989 (2 Suppl):33-50

32 Ekman P: BPH epidemiology and risk factors. Prostate 1989 (2 Suppl):23-31

33 Ohara-Nemoto Y, Strömstedt P-E, Dahlman-Wright K, Nemoto T, Gustafsson JÅ, Carlstedt-Duke J: The steroid-binding properties of recombinant glucocorticoid receptor: A putative role for heat shock protein hsp90. J Steroid Biochem Mol Biol 1990 (37):481-490

34 Schowalter DB, Sullivan WP, Maihle NJ et al: Characterization of progesterone receptor binding to the 90- and 70-kDa heat shock proteins. J Biol Chem 1991 (266):21165-21173

35 Cadepond F, Schweizer-Groyer G, Segard-Maurel I et al: Heat shock protein 90 as a critical factor in monitoring glucocorticoid receptor in a nonfunctional state. J Biol Chem 1991 (266):5834-5641

36 Picard D, Khursheed B, Garabedian MJ, Fortin MG, Lindquist S, Yamamoto KR: Reduced levels of hsp90 compromise steroid receptor action in vivo. Nature 1990 (348):166-168
37 Kumar V and Chambon P: The estrogen receptor binds tightly to its responsive element as a ligand-induced homodimer. Cell 1988 (55):145-156
38 Imperato-McGinley J, Guerrero L, Gautier T, Peterson RE: Steroid 5alpha-reductase deficiency in man: An inherited form of male pseudohermaphroditism. Science 1974 (186):1213-1215
39 Griffiths K, Akaza H, Eaton CL et al: Regulation of prostatic growth. In: Cockett ATK, Aso Y, Chatelain C, Denis L, Griffiths K, Khoury S, Murphy G (eds) Proceedings of the Second International Consultation on Benign Prostatic Hyperplasia (BPH), 1993. Publ SCI Paris, Paris 1994 pp 49-75
40 Isaacs JT: Antagonistic effect of androgen on prostatic cell death. Prostate 1984 (5):545-557
41 Bruchovsky N, Lesser B, van Doorn E, Craven S: Hormonal effects on cell proliferation in rat prostate. Vitam Horm 1975 (33):61-102
42 Beato M: Gene regulation by steroid hormones. Cell 1989 (56):335-344
43 Truss M and Beato M: Steroid hormone receptors: Interaction with deoxyribonucleic acid and transcription factors. Endocr Rev 1993 (14):459-479
44 Yamamoto KR: Steroid receptor regulated transcription of specific genes and gene networks. Ann Rev Genet 1985 (19):209-252
45 Gronemeyer H: Transcription activation by estrogen and progesterone receptors. Ann Rev Genet 1991 (25):89-123
46 Griffiths K, Akaza H, Eaton CL et al: Hormones, growth factors and benign prostatic hyperplasia (BPH). In: Cockett ATK, Aso Y, Chatelain C, Denis L, Griffiths K, Khoury S, Murphy G (eds) Proceedings of the First Consultation on Benign Prostatic Hyperplasia (BPH), 1991. Publ SCI Paris, Paris 1992 pp 25-49
47 Griffiths K, Davies P, Eaton CL, Harper ME, Turkes A, Peeling WB: Endocrine factors in the initiation, diagnosis, and treatment of prostatic cancer. In: Voigt KD and Knabbe C (eds) Endocrine Dependent Tumors. Raven Press, New York 1991 pp 83-130
48 Sporn MB and Roberts AB: Interactions of retinoids and transforming growth factor-ß in regulation of cell differentiation and proliferation. Mol Endocrinol 1991 (5):3-7
49 Sporn MB and Roberts AB: TGF-ß: Problems and prospects. Cell Regulation 1990 (1):875-882
50 Kyprianou N and Isaacs JT: Expression of transforming growth factor-ß in the rat ventral prostate during castration-induced programmed cell death. Mol Endocrinol 1989 (3):1515-1522
51 Wilding G, Valverius E, Knabbe C, Elmann EP: Role of transforming growth factor-α in human prostate cancer cell growth. Prostate 1989 (15):1-12
52 Cunha GR, Donjacour AA, Cooke PS et al: The endocrinology and developmental biology of the prostate. Endocr Rev 1987 (8):338-362
53 Franks LM, Riddle PN, Carbonell AW, Gey GO: A comparative study of the ultrastructure and lack of growth capacity of adult human prostate epithelium mechanically separated from its stroma. J Pathol 1970 (100):113-119
54 Krieg M, Bartsch W, Thomsen M, Voigt KD: Androgens and estrogens: Their interaction with stroma and epithelium of human benign prostatic hyperplasia and normal prostate. J Steroid Biochem 1983 (19):155-161
55 Lubrano C, Sciarra F, Spera G et al: Immunoreactive EGF in human benign prostatic hyperplasia: Relationships with androgen and estrogen receptors. J Steroid Biochem Mol Biol 1992 (41):683-687
56 St-Arnaud R, Poyet P, Walker P, Labrie F: Androgens modulate epidermal growth factor levels in the rat ventral prostate. Mol Cell Endocrinol 1988 (56): 21-27
57 Gregory H, Willshire IR, Kavanagh JP, Blacklock NJ, Chowdury S, Richards RC: Urogastrone-epidermal growth factor concentrations in prostatic fluid of normal individuals and patients with benign prostatic hypertrophy. Clin Sci 1986 (70):359-363
58 Maddy SQ, Chisholm GD, Hawkins RA, Habib FK: Localization of epidermal growth factor receptors in the human prostate by biochemical and immunocytochemical methods. J Endocrinol 1987 (113): 147-153
59 Davies P and Eaton CL: Binding of epidermal growth factor by human normal, hypertrophic and carcinomatous prostate. Prostate 1989 (14):123-132
60 Kabalin JN, Peehl DM, Stamey TA: Clonal growth of human prostatic epithelial cells is stimulated by fibroblasts. Prostate 1989 (14):251-263
61 Eaton CL: Growth factors, oncogenes and prostate cancer. Rev Endocrine Related Cancer 1992 (40): 5-12
62 Yan G, Fukabori Y, Nikolaropoulos S, Wang F, McKeehan WL: Heparin-binding keratinocyte growth factor is a candidate stromal to epithelial cell andromedin. Mol Endocrinol 1992 (6):2123-2128
63 Davies P, Eaton CL, France TD, Phillips MEA: Growth factor receptors and oncogene expression in prostate cells. Am J Clin Oncol 1988 (11 Suppl): S1-S7
64 Logan A and Hill DJ: Bioavailability: Is this a key event in regulating the actions of peptide growth factors? J Endocrinol 1992 (134):157-161
65 Cohen P, Peehl DM, Rosenfield RG. In: Proceedings of the International Symposium on Biology of Prostate Growth. Bethesda 1992 (in press)
66 Martinoli MG and Pelletier G: Dihydrotestosterone (DHT) regulation of insulin-like growth factor II mRNA in neonatal rats. Peptides 1991 (12):1267-1271
67 Cohen P, Peehl DM, Lamson G, Rosenfield RG: Insulin-like growth factors (IGFs), IGF receptors, and IGF-binding proteins in primary cultures of prostate epithelial cells. J Clin Endocrinol Metab 1991 (73):401-407
68 Cohen P, Graves HC, Peehl DM, Kamerai M, Giudice LC, Rosenfield RG: Prostate-specific antigen (PSA) is an insulin-like growth factor binding protein-3 protease found in seminal plasma. J Clin Endocrinol Metab 1992 (75):1046-1053
69 Muller WJ, Lee FS, Dickson C, Peters G, Pattengale P, Leder P: The int-2-gene product acts as an

epithelial growth factor in transgenic mice. EMBO J 1990 (9):907-913

70 Chaproniere DM and McKeehan WL: Serial culture of single adult human prostatic epithelial cells in serum-free medium containing low calcium and a new growth factor from bovine brain. Cancer Res 1986 (46):819-824

71 Finch PW, Rubin JS, Miki T, Ron D, Aaronson SA: Human KGF is FGF-related with properties of a paracrine effector of epithelial cell growth. Science 1989 (245):752-755

72 Miki T, Bottaro DP, Fleming TP: Determination of ligand-binding specificity by alternative splicing: Two distinct growth factor receptors encoded by a single gene. Proc Natl Acad Sci USA 1992 (89): 246-250

73 Mansson P-E, Adams P, Kan M, McKeehan WL: Heparin-binding growth factor gene expression and receptor characteristics in normal rat prostate and two transplantable rat prostate tumors. Cancer Res 1989 (49):2485-2494

74 Story MT, Livingstone B, Baeten L et al: Cultured human prostate-derived fibroblasts produce a factor that stimulates their growth with properties indistinguishable from basic fibroblast growth factor. Prostate 1989 (15):355-365

75 Hou J, Kan M, McKeehan K, McBride G, Adams P, McKeehan WL: Fibroblast growth factor receptors from liver vary in three structural domains. Science 1991 (251):665-668

76 Jaye M, Schlessinger J, Dionne CA: Fibroblast growth factor receptor tyrosine kinases: Molecular analysis and signal transduction. Biochim Biophys Acta 1992 (1135):185-199

77 Kan M, DiSorbo D, Hou J, Hoshi H, Mansson PE, McKeehan WL: High and low affinity binding of heparin-binding growth factor to a 130-kDa receptor correlates with stimulation and inhibition of growth of a differentiated human hepatoma cell. J Biol Chem 1988 (263):11306-11313

78 Kan M, Huang J, Mansson P-E, Yasumitsu H, Carr B, McKeehan WL: Heparin-binding growth factor type 1 (acidic fibroblast growth factor): A potential biphasic autocrine and paracrine regulation of hepatocyte regeneration. Proc Natl Acad Sci USA 1989 (86):7432-7436

79 Yan G, Wang F, Fukabori Y, Sussman D, Hou J, McKeehan WL: Expression and transforming activity of a variant of the heparin-binding fibroblast growth factor receptor (flg) gene resulting from splicing of the alpha exon at an alternate 3'-acceptor site. Biochem Biophys Res Commun 1992 (183): 423-430

80 Xu J, Nakahara M, Crabb JW et al: Expression and immunochemical analysis of rat and human fibroblast growth factor receptor (flg) isoforms. J Biol Chem 1992 (267):17992-17803

81 Sherwood ER, Fong C-J, Lee C, Kozlowski JM: Basic fibroblast growth factor: A potential mediator of stromal growth in the human prostate. Endocrinology 1992 (130):2955-2963

82 Story MT, Baeten LA, Molter MA, Lawson RK: Influence of androgen and transforming growth factor beta on basic fibroblast growth factor levels in human prostate-derived fibroblast cell cultures. J Urol 1990 (143 Suppl):abstract 211

83 Lee C, Sensibar JA, Dudek SM, Hiipakka RA, Liao S: Prostatic ductal system in rats: Regional variation in morphological and functional activities. Biol Reprod 1990 (43):1079-1086

84 Rouleau M, Léger J, Tenniswood M: Ductal heterogeneity of cytokeratins, gene expression, and cell death in the rat ventral prostate. Mol Endocrinol 1990 (4):2003-2013

85 Sugimura Y, Cunha GR, Donjacour AA: Morphogenesis of ductal networks in the mouse prostate. Biol Reprod 1986 (34):961-971

86 Berredge MJ: Inositol triphosphates and diacyl glycerol: Two interacting second messengers. Ann Rev Biochem 1987 (56):159-193

87 Bishop JM: Inositol triphosphate and diacylglycerol: Two interacting second messengers. Ann Rev Biochem 1983 (52):301-354

88 Weinberg RA: The action of oncogenes in the cytoplasm and nucleus. Science 1983 (230):770-776

89 Katz AE, Benson MC, Wise GJ et al: Gene activity during the early phase of androgen-stimulated rat prostate regrowth. Cancer Res 1989 (49):5889-5894

90 Davies P and Eaton CL: Regulation of prostate growth. J Endocrinol 1991 (131):5-17

91 Curran T, Bravo R, Müller R: Transient induction of c-fos and c-myc is an immediate consequence of growth factor stimulation. Cancer Surv 1985 (4): 655-681

92 Jones N: Transcriptional regulation by dimerization: Two sides to an incestuous relationship. Cell 1990 (61):9-11

93 Landschultz WH, Johnson PF, McKnight SL: The leucine zipper: A hypothetical structure common to a new class of DNA binding proteins. Science 1988 (240):1759-1764

94 Marx JL: The fos gene as 'master switch'. Science 1987 (237):854-856

95 Klein G: The approaching era of the tumour suppressor genes. Science 1987 (238):1539-1545

96 Huang H-JS, Yee J-K, Shew J-Y et al: Suppression of the neoplastic phenotype by replacement of the RB gene in human cancer cells. Science 1988 (242):1563-1566

97 Isaacs WB and Carter BS: Genetic changes associated with prostate cancer in humans. Cancer Surv 1991 (11):15-24

98 Denis L: Prostate cancer: Primary hormonal treatment. Cancer 1993 (71):1050-1058

99 Boyle P, Alexander FE, Standaert B, Denis L: Screening for prostate cancer. In: Henry W and Kirby R (eds) Recent Advances in Urology. Churchill-Livingstone, Edinburgh 1995 (in press)

100 Schroeder FH and Boyle P: Screening for prostate cancer: Necessary or nonsense? Eur J Cancer 1993 (29A):656-661

101 Morton RA, Steiner MS, Walsh PC: Cancer control following anatomical radical prostatectomy: An interim report. J Urol 1991 (145):1197-1200

102 Bagshaw MA,Cox RS, Ray GR: Status of radiation treatment of prostate cancer at Stanford University. NCI Monogr 1988 (7):47-60

103 Griffiths K, Eaton CL, Harper ME, Turkes A, Peeling WB: Endocrine aspects of prostate cancer. Rev Endocrine-Related Cancer 1993 (42):5-22
104 Gormley G, Ferguson D, Lieber M et al: Effect of finasteride on patients with elevated PSA following radical prostatectomy for prostate cancer. J Urol 1993 (149 Suppl): abstract 255
105 Baserga R, Porcu P, Sell C: Onogenes, growth factors and control of the cell cycle. Cancer Surv 1993 (16):201-213
106 Evans RM: The steroid and thyroid hormone receptor superfamily. Science 1988 (240):889-895
107 Bishop JM: The molecular genetics of cancer. Science 1987 (235):305-311
108 Varmus H and Bishop JM: Introduction. Cancer Surv 1986 (5):153-158
109 Sager R: Tumor suppressor genes: The puzzle and the promise. Science 1989 (246):1406-1412
110 Diamond MI, Miner JN, Yoshinaga SK, Yamamoto KR: Transcription factor interactions: Selections of positive or negative regulation from a single DNA element. Science 1990 (249):1266-1272
111 Roche PJ, Hoare SA, Parker MG: A consensus DNA-binding site for the androgen receptor. Mol Endocrinol 1992 (6):2229-2235
112 Slater EP, Redeuilh G, Beato M: Hormonal regulation of vitellogenin genes: An estrogen-responsive element in the xenopus A2 gene and a multihormonal regulatory region in the chicken II gene. Mol Endocrinol 1991 (5):386-396
113 Chang C, Kokontis J, Liao S: Molecular cloning of human and rat complementary DNA encoding androgen receptors. Science 1988 (240):324-326
114 Tan J, Joseph DR, Quarmby VE et al: The rat androgen receptor: Primary structure, autoregulation of its messenger ribonucleic acid, and immunocytochemical localization of the receptor protein. Mol Endocrinol 1988 (2):1276-1285
115 Lubahn DB, Joseph DR, Sar M et al: The human androgen receptor: Complementary deoxyribonucleic acid cloning, sequence analysis and gene expression in prostate. Mol Endocrinol 1988 (2):1265-1275
116 Lubahn DB, Joseph DR, Sullivan PM, Willard HF, French FS, Wilson EM: Cloning of human androgen receptor complementary DNA and localization to the X chromosome. Science 1988 (240):327-330
117 Trapman J, Klaassen P, Kuiper GGJM et al: Cloning, structure and expression of a cDNA encoding the human androgen receptor. Biochem Biophys Res Commun 1988 (153):241-248
118 van Laar JH, Bolt-de-Vries J, Voorhorst-Ogink MM, Brinkmann AO: The human androgen receptor is a 110 kDa protein. Mol Cell Endocrinol 1989 (63):39-44
119 Kuiper GGJM, Faber PW, van Rooij HCJ, van der Korput JAGM, Ris-Stalpers C, Klaassen P, Trapman J, Brinkman AO: Structural organization of the human androgen receptor gene. J Mol Endocrinol 1989 (2):R1-R4
120 Huckaby CS, Conneely OM, Beattie WG, Dobson ADW, Tsai M-J, O'Malley BW: Structure of the chromosomal chicken progesterone receptor gene. Proc Natl Acad Sci USA 1987 (84):8380-8384
121 Ponglikitmongkol M, Green S, Chambon P: Genomic organization of the human oestrogen receptor gene. EMBO J 1988 (7):3385-3388
122 Faber PW, Kuiper GGJM, van Rooij HCJ, van der Korput JAGM, Brinkmann AO, Trapman J: The N-terminal domain of the human androgen receptor is encoded by one, large exon. Mol Cell Endocrinol 1989 (61):257-262
123 Evans RM and Hollenberg SM: Zinc fingers: Gilt by association. Cell 1988 (52):1-3
124 Green S and Chambon P: Nuclear receptors enhance our understanding of transcription regulation. Trend Genet 1988 (4):309-314
125 Howard KJ, Holley SJ, Yamamoto KR, Distelhorst CW: Mapping the hsp90 binding region of the glucocorticoid receptor. J Biol Chem. 1990 (265):11928-11935
126 Eriksson P and Wrange Ö: Protein-protein contacts in the glucocorticoid receptor homodimer influence its DNA binding properties. J Biol Chem 1990 (265):3535-3542
127 Schwabe JWR and Rhodes D: Beyond zinc fingers: Steroid hormone receptors have a novel structural motif for DNA recognition. Trends Biochem Sci 1991 (16):291-296
128 Fawell SE, Lees JA, White R, Parker MG: Characterization and colocalization of steroid binding and dimerization activities in the mouse estrogen receptor. Cell 1990 (60):953-962
129 Hollenberg SM and Evans RM: Multiple and cooperative trans-activation domains of the human glucocorticoid receptor. Cell 1988 (55):899-906
130 Giguère V, Hollenberg SM, Rosenfeld MG, Evans RM: Functional domains of the human glucocorticoid receptor. Cell 1986 (46):645-652
131 Kumar V, Green S, Stack G, Berry M, Jin J-R, Chambon P: Functional domains of the human estrogen receptor. Cell 1987 (51):941-951
132 Webster NJG, Green S, Jin JR, Chambon P: The hormone-binding domains of the estrogen and glucocorticoid receptors contain an inducible transcription activation function. Cell 1988 (54):199-207
133 Klein-Hitpass L, Ryffel GU, Heitlinger E, Cato ACB: A 13 bp palindrome is a functional estrogen responsive element and interacts specifically with estrogen receptor. Nucleic Acids Res 1988 (16): 647-663
134 Denison SH, Sands A, Tindall DJ: A tyrosine aminotransferase glucocorticoid response element also mediates androgen enhancement of gene expression. Endocrinology 1989 (124):1091-1093
135 Cato ACB, Henderson D, Ponta H: The hormone response element of the mouse mammary tumour virus DNA mediates the progestin and androgen induction of transcription in the proviral long terminal repeat region. EMBO J 1987 (6):363-368
136 Ham J, Thomson A, Needham M, Webb P, Parker MG: Characterization of response elements for androgens, glucocorticoids and progestins in mouse mammary tumour virus. Nucleic Acids Res 1988 (16):5263-5276
137 Rushmere NK, Parker MG, Davies P: Androgen receptor-binding regions of an androgen-responsive gene. Mol Cell Endocrinol 1987 (51):259-265

138 Heyns W and De Moor P: Prostatic binding protein: A steroid binding protein secreted by rat prostate. Eur J Biochem 1977 (78):221-230

139 Claessens F, Rushmere NK, Davies P, Celis L, Peeters B, Rombauts WA: Sequence-specific binding of androgen-receptor complexes to prostatic binding protein genes. Mol Cell Endocrinol 1990 (74):203-212

140 Medici N, Nigro V, Abbondanza C, Moncharmont B, Molinari AM, Puca GA: In vitro binding of the purified hormone-binding subunit of the estrogen receptor to oligonucleotides containing natural or modified sequences of an estrogen-responsive element. Mol Endocrinol 1991 (5):555-563

141 Berry M, Nunez A-M, Chambon P: Estrogen-responsive element of the human pS2 gene is an imperfectly palindromic sequence. Proc Natl Acad Sci USA 1989 (86):1218-1222

142 Tsai SY, Tsai M-J, O'Malley BW: Cooperative binding of steroid hormone receptors contributes to transcriptional synergism at target enhancer elements. Cell 1989 (57):443-448

143 Schüle R, Muller M, Kaltschmidt C, Renkawitz R: Many transcription factors interact synergistically with steroid receptors. Science 1988 (242):1418-1420

144 Shemshedini L, Knauthe R, Sassone-Corsi P, Pornon A, Gronemeyer H: Cell-specific inhibitory and stimulatory effects of fos and jun on transcription activation by nuclear receptors. EMBO J 1991 (10): 3839-3849

145 Sabbah M, Le Ricousse S, Redeuilh G, Baulieu E-E: Estrogen receptor-induced binding of the xenopus vitellogenin A2 gene hormone response element. Biochem Biophys Res Commun 1992 (185): 944-952

146 Nardulli AM and Shapiro DJ: Binding of the estrogen receptor DNA-binding domain to the estrogen response element induces DNA binding. Mol Cell Biol 1992 (12):2037-2042

147 Klock G, Strähle U, Schütz G: Oestrogen and glucocorticoid responsive elements are closely related but distinct. Nature 1987 (329):734-736

148 Truss M, Chalepakis G, Slater EP, Mader S, Beato M: Functional interaction of hybrid response elements with wild-type and mutant steroid hormone receptors. Mol Cell Biol 1991 (11):3247-3258

149 Truss M, Chalepakis G, Beato M: Contacts between steroid hormone receptors and thymines in DNA: An interference method. Proc Natl Acad Sci USA 1990 (87):7180-7184

150 Martinez E, Givel F, Wahli W: The estrogen-responsive element as an inducible enhancer: DNA sequence requirements and conversion to a glucocorticoid-responsive element. EMBO J 1987 (6): 3719-3727

151 Freedman LP: Anatomy of the steroid receptor zinc finger region. Endocr Rev 1992 (13):129-145

152 Luisi BF, Xu WX, Otwinowski Z, Freedman LP, Yamamoto KR, Sigler PB: Crystallographic analysis of the interaction of the glucocorticoid receptor with DNA. Nature 1991 (352):497-505

153 Barbacid M: Ras Genes. Ann Rev Biochem 1987 (56):779-827

154 Gilman AG: G proteins: Transducers of receptor-generated signals. Ann Rev Biochem 1987 (56): 615-649

155 Cole MD: The myc oncogene: Its role in transformation and differentiation. Ann Rev Genet 1986 (20):361-384

156 Rijnders AWM, van der Korput JAGM, van Steenbrugge GJ, Romijn JC, Trapman J: Expression of cellular oncogenes in human prostatic carcinoma cell lines. Biochem Biophys Res Commun 1985 (132):548-554

157 Phillips MEA, Ferro MA, Smith PJB, Davies P: Intranuclear androgen receptor deployment and protooncogene expression in human diseased prostate. Urol Int 1987 (42):115-119

158 Treiger B and Isaacs JT: Expression of a transfected v-Harvey-«it»ras«rt» oncogene in a Dunning rat prostate adenocarcinoma and the development of high metastatic ability. J Urol 1988 (140):1580-1586

159 Thompson TC, Kadmon D, Timme TL et al: Experimental oncogene induced prostate cancer. Cancer Surv 1991 (11):55-71

160 Buttyan R, Sawczuk IS, Benson MC, Siegal JD, Olsson CA: Enhanced expression of the c-myc protooncogene in high-grade human prostate cancers. Prostate 1987 (11):327-337

161 Yan G, Fukabori Y, McBride G, Nikolaropolous S, McKeehan WL: Exon switching and activation of stromal and embryonic fibroblast growth factor (FGF)-FGF receptor genes in prostate epithelial cells accompany stromal independence and malignancy. Mol Cell Biol 1993 (13):4513-4522

162 Shi E, Kan M, Xu J, Wang F, Hou J, McKeehan WL: Control of fibroblast growth factor receptor kinase signal transduction by heterodimerization of combinatorial splice variants. Mol Cell Biol 1993 (13):3907-3918

163 Postel EH, Berberich SJ, Flint SJ, Ferrone CA: Human c-myc transcription factor PuF identified as nm23-H2 nucleoside diphosphate kinase, a candidate suppressor of tumor metastasis. Science 1993 (261):478-480

164 Steeg PS, Bevilacqua G, Kopper L et al: Evidence for a novel gene associated with low tumor metastatic potential. JNCI 1988 (80):200-204

165 Leone A, Flatow U, van Houtte K, Steeg PS: Transfection of human nm23-H1 into the human MDA-MB-435 breast carcinoma cell line: Effects on tumor metastatic potential, colonization and enzymatic activity. Oncogene 1993 (8):2325-2333

166 Stahl JA, Leone A, Rosengard AM: Identification of a second human nm23 gene, nm23-H2. Cancer Res 1991 (51):445-449

167 Black DM, Nicolai H, Borrow J, Solomon E: A somatic cell hybrid map of the long arm of human chromosome 17, containing the familial breast cancer locus (BRCA1). Am J Hum Genet 1993 (52):702-710

168 Weisz A and Rosales R: Identification of an estrogen response element upstream of the human c-fos gene that binds the estrogen receptor and the AP-1 transcription factor. Nucleic Acids Res 1990 (18): 5097-5106

169 Weisz A, Cicatiello L, Persico E, Scalona M, Bresciani F: Estrogen stimulates transcription of c-jun protooncogene. Mol Endocrinol 1990 (4):1041-1050
170 Schulze H and Isaacs JT: Biology and therapy of prostatic cancer. Cancer Surv 1986 (5):487-503
171 King RJB: Progression from steroid sensitive to insensitive state in breast tumours. Cancer Surv 1992 (14):131-146
172 French FS, Lubahn DB, Brown TR et al: Rec Prog Hormone Res 1990 (46):1-42
173 Veldscholte J, Ris-Stalpers C, Kuiper GGJM et al: A mutation in the ligand binding domain of the androgen receptor of human LNCaP cells affects steroid binding characteristics and response to anti-androgens. Biochem Biophys Res Commun 1990 (173):534-540
174 Evans BAJ, Harper ME, Daniells CE et al: Low incidence of androgen receptor gene mutations in human prostatic tumors using single strand conformation polymorphism analysis. Prostate 1995 (in press)
175 Wakeling AE, Furr BJA, Glen AT, Hughes LR: Receptor binding and biological activity of steroidal and nonsteroidal antiandrogens. J Steroid Biochem 1981 (15):355-359
176 Kelly WK and Scher HI: Prostate specific antigen decline after antiandrogen withdrawal: The flutamide withdrawal syndrome. J Urol 1993 (149): 607-609
177 Nicholson RI and Griffiths K: The biochemistry of tamoxifen action. In: Thomas JA and Singhal RL (eds) Advances in Sex Hormone Research. Urban & Schwarzenberg, Baltimore/Munich 1980 pp 119-152
178 Fawell SE, White R, Hoare S, Sydenham M, Page M, Parker MG: Inhibition of estrogen receptor-DNA binding by the 'pure' antiestrogen ICI 164,384 appears to be mediated by impaired receptor dimerization. Proc Natl Acad Sci USA 1990 (87):6883-6887
179 Bowler J, Lilley TJ, Pittam JD, Wakeling AE: Novel steroidal pure antiestrogens. Steroids 1989 (54): 71-99

Pharmacology of Cyproterone Acetate - A Short Review

Friedmund Neumann

Ernst Schering Research Foundation, Müllerstrasse 178, 13342 Berlin, Germany

Cyproterone acetate (CPA) was the first antiandrogen to be used in clinical practice. The antiandrogenic activity was discovered in 1962/1963 - 30 years ago. But the term "antiandrogen" was not really new [for review see 1].
Most compounds which were labelled "antiandrogens" before 1962 were simply too weak. Many were only effective in certain species, in chickens but not in mammals, for instance, others were only antiandrogenic at certain dose levels but had an androgenic effect when given at higher doses (agonistic effects). Yet other substances were too toxic and had to be excluded from clinical trials altogether. No one had any clear idea as to what the structure of a potent androgen antagonist would look like.
No antiandrogen was available for clinical use when Dorfman [1] wrote the chapter on antiandrogens in his book *Methods in Hormone Research*. It was also he who mentioned potential indications for antiandrogens, because it had long been assumed that certain diseases and conditions are induced or unfavourably influenced by androgens.
The following indications were mentioned: "Systemically active compounds may be of enormous benefit for women suffering from certain types of hirsutism and men suffering from androgen-dependent tumours. Local use of antiandrogenic compounds could also be of use in women with hypertrichosis, in prevention of certain types of male baldness, for the inhibition of facial hair growth in women, and for the treatment and/or prevention of acne in young men and women."
And what has been achieved? There are still no antiandrogenic preparations available for local use (topical application), although there is a certain need for them. Because of the effects of antiandrogens on, for example, spermatogenesis, libido and potency, the systemic treatment of men with acne problems or baldness is not possible. The ideal solution would be a topically active antiandrogen without systemic side-effects, but this problem has not yet been solved.
Dorfman also mentioned hypertrichosis but, since androgens are not involved in the aetiology of this disorder, a therapeutic effect of antiandrogens is also unlikely.
Of the indications for antiandrogens mentioned by Dorfman only hirsutism, acne and tumours of the prostate (prostatic carcinoma) have been realised. There are, however, some other indications which were not mentioned but for which CPA is used, for example hypersexuality and precocious puberty.
It was again Dorfman [2] who offered a definition of antiandrogens: "Antiandrogens are substances which prevent androgens from expressing their activity at target sites. The inhibitory effect of these substances, therefore, would be differentiated from compounds which decrease the synthesis and/or release of hypothalamic (releasing factors) and anterior pituitary hormones (gonadotrophins, particularly luteinising hormone) and materials which act directly on the gonads to inhibit biosynthesis and/or secretion of androgens."
This definition is fulfilled only by so-called pure antiandrogens (some also call them "direct acting" antiandrogens) such as flutamide, nilutamide and Casodex but not by CPA, chlormadinone acetate and megoestrol acetate, which are also quite potent progestogens. For most indications this is an advantage rather than a disadvantage as compared with pure antiandrogens.
Since the most prominent representatives of the class of pure antiandrogens, namely flu-

Table 1. Indications for cyproterone acetate (CPA) containing preparations

Indication	Preparation used
Androgenisation in women	
acne seborrhoea moderate hirsutism	Diane-35® (2 mg cyproterone acetate + 35 µg ethinyloestradiol)
severe hirsutism androgenic alopecia	50-100 mg CPA during the first 10 days of the cycle, Diane-35® for 21 days or non-stop treatment with CPA alone in postmenopausal or hysterectomised patients or 300 mg CPA i.m. on the first day of the cycle, Diane-35® for 21 days
Prostatic carcinoma	depending on whether the patient is orchidectomised or not 100-300 mg CPA/day or 300 mg CPA i.m. once a week
Precocious puberty	100-300 mg CPA/m^2 body area
Hypersexuality (reduction of sex drive in sexual deviations)	200-300 mg CPA/day or 300 mg CPA i.m. every 10 or 14 days

tamide, nilutamide and Casodex, have a non-steroidal structure in common, whereas CPA, chlormadinone acetate and megoestrol acetate are steroidal compounds, both classes are usually differentiated by the terms "non-steroidal" or "steroidal" antiandrogens.

Until now there is only one indication for non-steroidal antiandrogens, namely, prostate carcinoma. Table 1 shows the indications for CPA-containing preparations.

Discovery of CPA

At the beginning of the 1960s, we had the task of synthesising and developing oral active and better tolerable progestogens and androgens. One indication for progestogens at that time was "threatened abortion".

All of the oral active progestogens available then were testosterone derivatives. Nevertheless, these compounds have been used to treat pregnant women, especially in the United States. As could be expected, the daughters of women who had been treated with these types of progestogens showed signs of virilisation, for instance fusion of the labioscrotal folds or hypertrophy of the clitoris. Any new progestogen for the mentioned indication (threatened abortion) had to be free of the virilising side-effects of testosterone derivatives. Our chemists sought to modify the progesterone molecule, the natural corpus luteum hormone, in the hope of finding an oral active derivative without virilising (androgenic) side-effects. Progesterone itself is orally inactive; it is metabolised in several positions by hydroxylases, reductases and dehydrogenases.

To inhibit the metabolism of progesterone by enzymes, space-filling substituents were incorporated into the steroid molecule. The result of these efforts was CPA, a hydroxyprogesterone derivative. At that time, CPA was the most potent progestogen of all hydroxyprogesterone derivatives (Fig. 1) [3]. The problem appeared to be solved, because due to the chemical structure of CPA it was very unlikely that this compound could possess androgenic (virilising) properties. Nevertheless, to be on the safe side a relevant test was performed. Female rats were treated during the last quarter of pregnancy and the fetuses were removed and examined at about term.

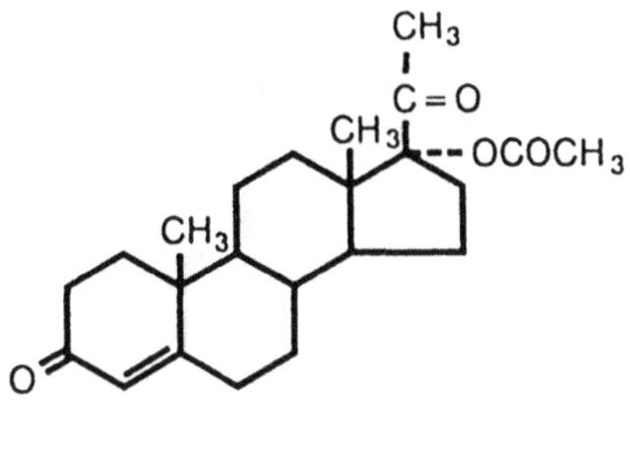

17α – Hydroprogesterone acetate
(A)

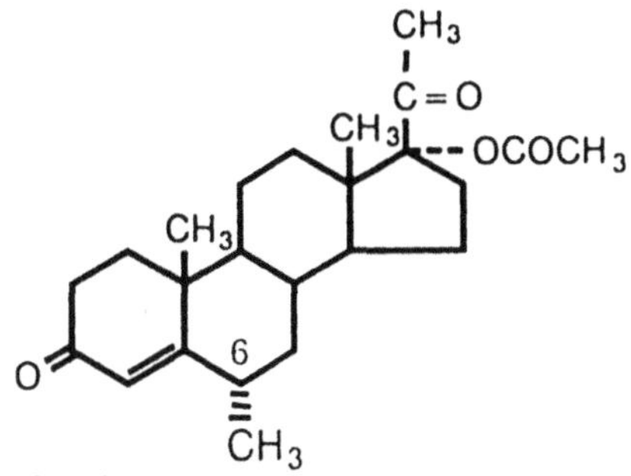

Medroxyprogesterone acetate
(B)

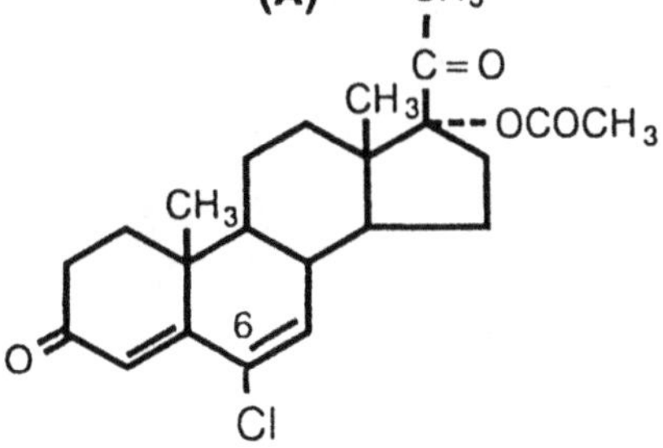

Chlormadinone acetate
(C)

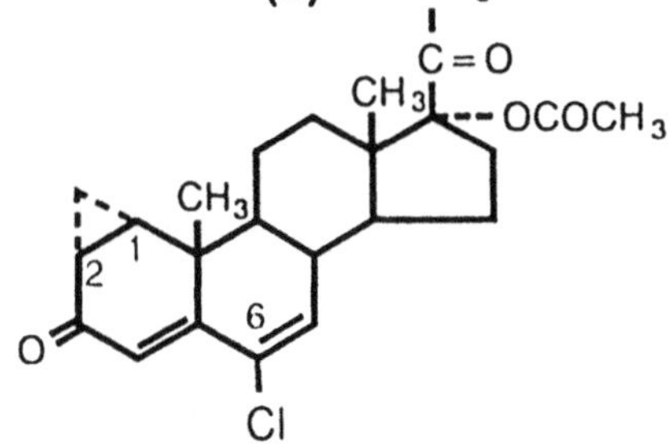

Cyproterone acetate
(D)

Relative oral progestational activity
(A) = 1 (B) = 100 (C) = 400 (D) = 1200

Fig. 1. Highly active progestational derivatives of 17-acetoxyprogesterone

Usually it is very easy to distinguish between female and male fetuses by inspection of the external genitalia. This was not possible with fetuses from this experiment. It appeared that only female fetuses were present. As the 20th female fetus had been counted, it became apparent that this was no coincidence. CPA must have had a very special effect never seen with any other progestogen or hormone before.
More detailed examination revealed that about 50% of the fetuses of treated mothers were males. This form of intersexuality had not been seen before in animals, but closely resembled a specific form of intersexuality in humans called "testicular feminisation" or "hairless women" [4,5].
Figure 2 shows the result of the now almost historical experiment, namely serial sections through rat fetuses: a male, a female, and a male of a treated mother. In males of treated mothers, all steps of sexual differentiation that were assumed to be androgen-dependent did not occur, e.g. the perineum was just as narrow as in the female animal and the size and shape of the penis corresponded to those of a clitoris. A vagina was partially developed. All these effects were irreversible, as we showed later in different species, including dogs. In contrast to the term "virilisation", we called this phenomenon "feminisation".
The only possible cause of feminisation could be androgen deficiency. There were two possibilities: either CPA inhibited the androgen biosynthesis in the fetal testes or this compound inhibited the action of androgens in one way or another directly at the target organ level.
The following experiment proved the second theory to be correct (see Fig. 3). In this experiment, castrated mice were given testosterone propionate. The parameters used for androgenicity were seminal vesicle and prostate weights.
As can be seen, the prostate and seminal vesicle weights in castrated animals can be maintained by testosterone propionate. This effect was inhibited in a dose-dependent manner when CPA was given in addition. From the curve it is quite obvious that we are dealing with a competitive type of antagonism. This was the birthday of the first antiandrogen suitable for clinical use.

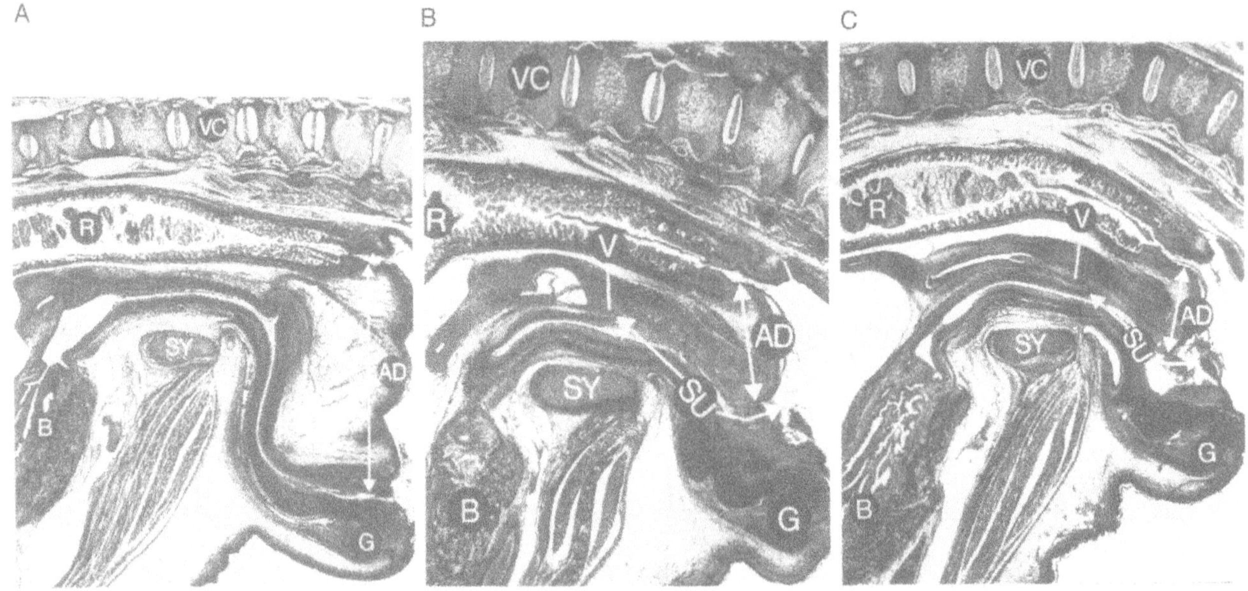

Fig. 2. Sagittal sections of rat fetuses on day 22 of fetal development
A Normal male fetus
B "Feminised" male fetus. The mother was treated with 10 mg of cyproterone acetate per day from day 17 to day 20 of gestation
C Normal female fetus
B = urinary bladder, AD = anogenital distance, R = rectum, SU = urogenital sinus, G = glans penis or clitoris, respectively, SY = symphysis pelvis, V = vagina, VC = vertebral column
Magnification: x 9
Staining: Haematoxylin Eosin

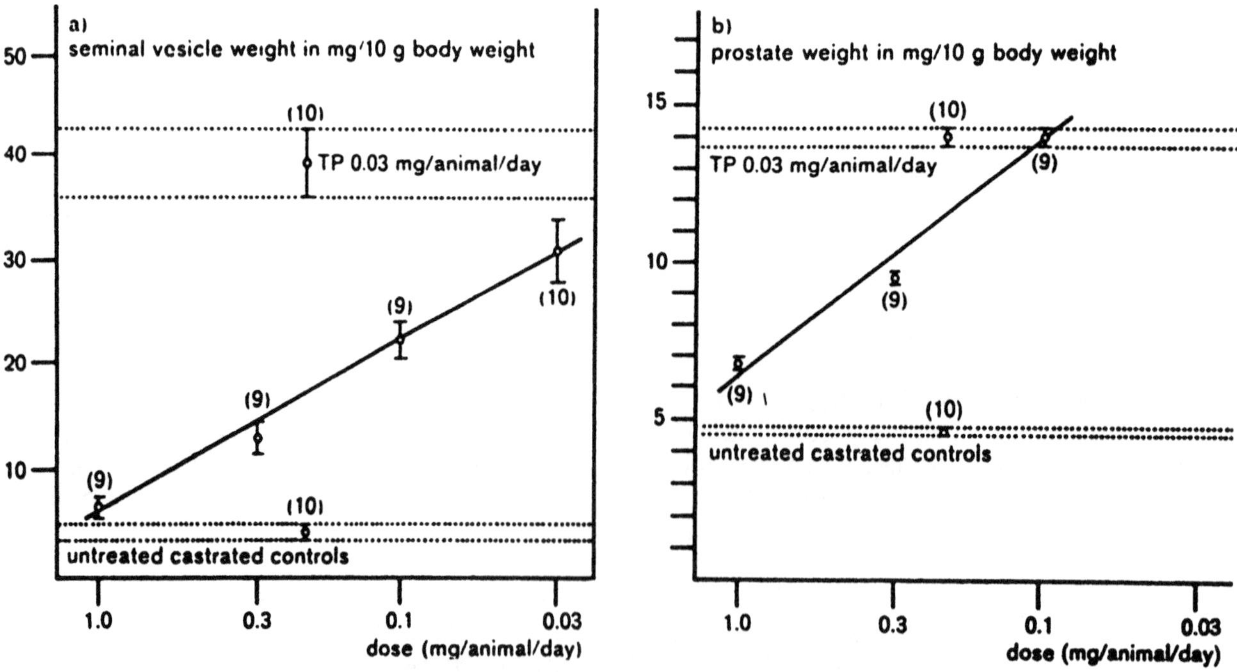

Fig. 3. Inhibition of action of 0.03 mg testosterone propionate (TP) by cyproterone acetate (examined in adult male castrated mice treated for 7 days subcutaneously)
Standard error
(x) Number of animals

Mechanism of Action

The mechanism of action of androgens and of steroids in general was unknown at that time (1962/1963). The general belief was that steroid hormones act by enzyme activation [6]. The receptor concept developed by Jensen and Jacobson [7] was not accepted until the mid sixties. It is interesting that in experiments which clarified the molecular mechanism of action of androgens as described by Fang and Liao [8], CPA and cyproterone (the free alcohol, free of progestational activities and therefore by definition a pure antiandrogen) were used to prove the specificity of the receptor concept.
In this historical experiment, Fang and Liao treated rats with radioactive testosterone. They were then able to identify a dihydrotestosterone protein complex (hormone receptor complex) in prostate nuclei by sucrose gradient centrifugation. If CPA or cyproterone were given together with testosterone, then the hormone receptor complex was no longer detectable. From this experiment it was postulated that antiandrogens inhibit the translocation of the cytosolic hormone receptor complex into the nucleus.
There is some agreement now that antiandrogens compete with androgens for nuclear receptor sites. It is questionable whether a receptor protein exists in the cytoplasm. Anyhow, antiandrogens reduce the amount of functionally active androgen receptors in the nuclei of target cells.

Pharmacokinetics [9-12]

CPA is completely absorbed following oral administration, without being subject to a first-pass effect. It reaches the major circulation in unchanged form and is therefore almost 100% bioavailable. Maximal substance levels are reached 3 to 4 hours after administration. The greatest part of CPA is eliminated via the kidneys and bile in the form of non-conjugated metabolites. About 30% of the urinary metabolites and 50% to 60% of the metabolic products in the bile are conjugated with glucuronic acid. About 10% of the biliary and urinary metabolites are in the form of sulphates. The main metabolite is 15ß-hydroxy-cyproterone-acetate. Approximately 30% of the metabolites are eliminated with the urine and 70% with the bile. The terminal half-life is about 30 to 40 hours. CPA does not accumulate. An equilibrium between administration and excretion is established after 8 to 10 days' use. With a half-life of almost 2 days a highly constant concentration is achieved in target tissues for androgens (and antiandrogens).
The administration of the depot (300 mg/ampoule) leads after 2 to 3 days to maximal substance levels of about 300 to 400 ng/ml with a half-life of 4 days. An equilibrium is established after 4 injections (7-day intervals) at the latest.

Pharmacology

The pharmacology of CPA has been described in at least 150 articles and several book chapters by our group [for reviews see 13-19], and at least 300 to 500 articles have been published by other authors; in the latter CPA was used mainly as a tool in basic research.
In this short review only few data will be presented from pharmacological studies which were undertaken to establish the rational basis for the different indications. Those studies in which CPA was used as a tool in basic research will not be discussed [for reviews see 13,19-22].
CPA acts in all target organs for androgens and, in principle, exerts all functions which are governed or influenced by androgens under physiological or pathophysiological conditions. Some of these more or less sex-specific effects are listed in Table 2.
The first indication thought of for CPA was carcinoma of the prostate. We were convinced from the start that this antiandrogen would be superior to all other known methods of androgen deprivation in the palliative therapy of metastatic carcinoma of the prostate for two reasons: 1) the lower potential for side-effects as compared with oestrogens, and 2) the ability of CPA to eliminate the effects of androgens of both testicular and adrenal origin.
As mentioned above - and as will be shown later - CPA is also a highly potent progestin and, as such, inhibits gonadotrophin secretion (unlike pure antiandrogens such as flutamide). CPA is therefore unique in combining the two basic principles of androgen deprivation (dual

Table 2. Effects of cyproterone acetate on organs and functions

Organ system/function	Effect of cyproterone acetate
Accessory sexual glands	Atrophy, loss of secretory activity
Spermatogenesis	Inhibition
Libido and potency	Loss of libido (except in some rodents)
Puberty	Inhibition of onset of puberty
Male sexual differentiation	Feminisation
Longitudinal bone growth	Retardation
Bone maturation, ossification	Retardation
Sebaceous gland function	Inhibition

mechanism of action): 1) reduction of androgen biosynthesis, and 2) inhibition of androgenic activity at the cellular level.

Antiandrogenic Properties

Accessory Sexual Glands (Prostate, Seminal Vesicles)

It has been shown in a large number of pharmacological studies in different species that the effect of CPA - when given at high enough doses - is the same as that of surgical castration. Experiments in the dog revealed inhibition of both proliferative and secretory activity. All characteristic enzymes and constituents of the prostate, such as acid phosphatase, aminopeptidase and zinc, are reduced to castration levels [14,23-25].

As an example, Figure 4 shows the behaviour of acid phosphatase in the dog after 6 months' administration of CPA.

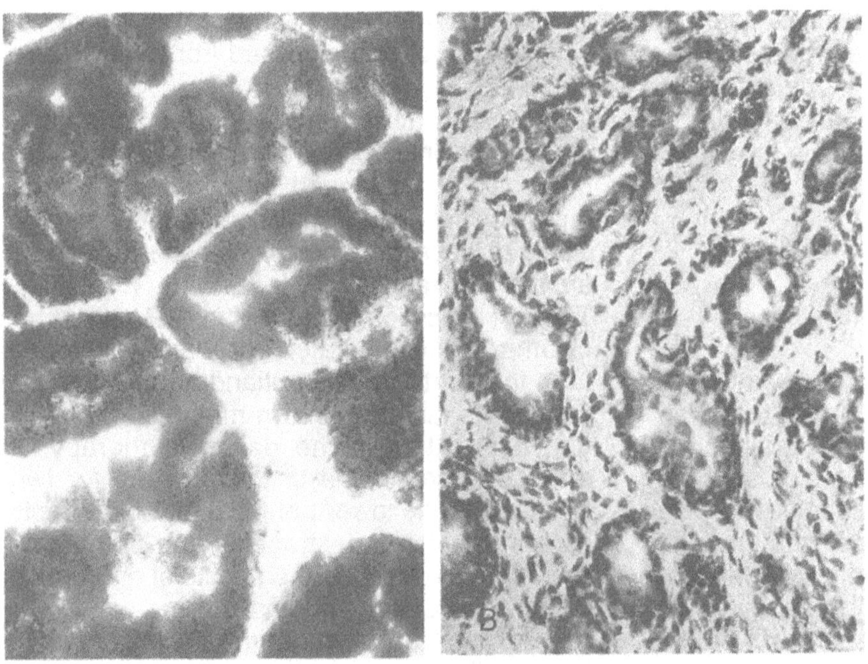

Fig. 4. Prostate of castrated dogs
A After 6 months of treatment with 3,17ß-androstanediol (25 mg weekly)
B After 6 months of treatment with 3,17ß-androstanediol (25 mg weekly) plus cyproterone acetate (600 mg weekly)
Magnification: approx. x 800. Staining: Acid phosphatase

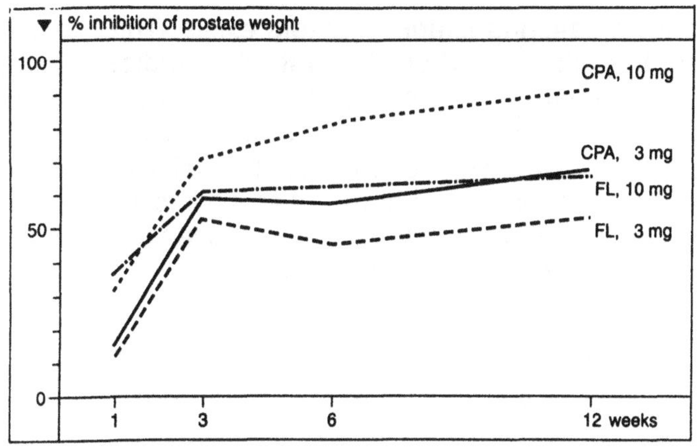

Fig. 5. Long-term effects of the antiandrogens cyproterone acetate (CPA) and flutamide (FL) on prostate weight in adult intact male rats

Antiandrogenic Potency of CPA and Flutamide

Pure antiandrogens (flutamide has been tested) are relatively more effective in castrated and androgen replaced animals than CPA. In intact animals, on the other hand, CPA is much more active. This is explained by the counterregulatory mechanisms by which pure antiandrogens stimulate testosterone biosynthesis in both experimental animals and men.

Animal experiments revealed that this counterregulatory effect of pure antiandrogens also influences the morphology of the hypothalamus, the pituitary, and the testes. Within the hypothalamus there is an increase in LHRH containing neurons. In the pituitary the gonadotrophin producing cells are increased in number and size. The consequence of increased LH secretion is Leydig cell hyperplasia in the testes [26].

It has been argued that, in sufficiently high concentrations, pure antiandrogens should be able to completely antagonise the effect of even high amounts of androgens at the receptor level [27]. That this is not the case has been shown in animal studies (Fig. 5). In contrast to the effect of CPA it is not possible, even with high doses of flutamide, to inhibit prostate weights of intact rats completely. This is an important difference between pure antiandrogens and steroidal antiandrogens, because the question is left open whether pure antiandrogens are suitable for monotherapy in prostate cancer patients, that is, whether they are as effective as other procedures of androgen withdrawal [26].

CPA in Combination with LHRH Agonists in the Initial Phase of Use

Twenty-four hours after a single treatment, the concentrations of both LH and testosterone were drastically increased in rats which had been treated with flutamide alone or with the combination LHRH agonist (lutrelin) plus flutamide. This increase, which is induced primarily by flutamide, did not occur in the group in which the animals had been treated with the combination lutrelin plus CPA.

The LH values in the groups treated with flutamide alone, lutrelin alone or flutamide plus lutrelin were still clearly elevated after a week, while - as under monotherapy with CPA - they were still within the control range, i.e., not stimulated by the additional treament with lutrelin, in animals treated with CPA plus lutrelin.

The LH values in the group treated with flutamide plus lutrelin were no longer elevated after 3 weeks. However, the LH values were definitively inhibited only in the group treated with 10 mg CPA plus lutrelin [28].

In human volunteers pretreatment with CPA reduced the initial increase in LH and testosterone induced by buserelin [28]. The inhibition of the LHRH-induced "biochemical flare-up" by pretreatment (one week) with CPA was confirmed in patients suffering from prostate cancer [29]. As a quite potent progestogen (see later), CPA does also inhibit the occurrence of hot flushes after orchidectomy or under treatment with LHRH analogues [30,31].

Clinical Dose-Finding Studies

It is difficult - if not impossible - to perform dose-finding studies in patients when no method for measuring tumour markers exists. This was the situation when the first pilot studies with CPA started. Animal data alone are not very helpful and the decrease in testosterone serum concentration does not tell the full truth because the main mechanism of action is competition with testosterone for receptor sites and this cannot be measured in humans.

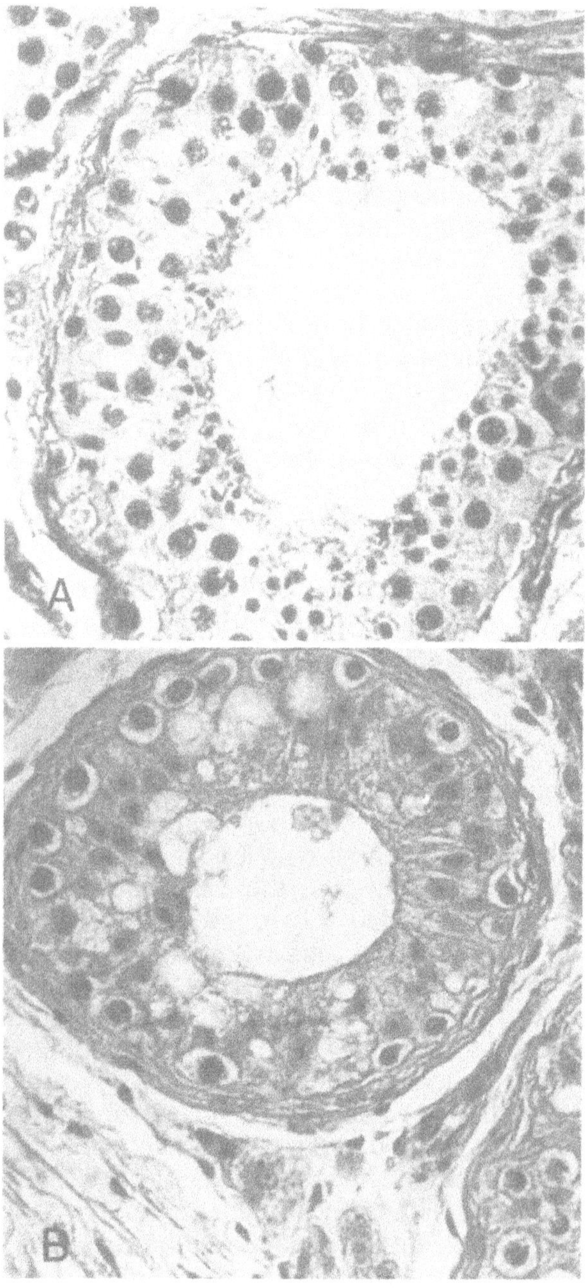

Fig. 6. Inhibition of spermatogenesis in man
(A) Before and (B) after approximately one year of treatment with cyproterone acetate (100 mg/daily p.o.)
Magnification: ca. x 250
Staining: Haematoxylin Eosin

Fortunately, we had at our disposal data from hypersexuals (sexual offenders) treated with different doses of CPA (suppression of sexual drive was the first indication). These data showed that with daily dosages of 100 mg the patients, or at least those who were still capable, achieved a so-called dry orgasm, that is, there was no ejaculate: the secretory activity of the accessory sex glands had ceased completely [for review see 32]. This resembles the effect of surgical castration.
The recommended dose for monotherapy with CPA is 200 to 300 mg/day. This is approximately 3 times as high as the dose that completely inhibits the secretory function of the "healthy" prostate. The recommended dose for combined therapy is 100 to 200 mg. This should be more than sufficient to inhibit the effect of adrenal androgens in orchidectomised patients or those treated with an LHRH-analogue.

Effect of CPA on Libido and Potency (Treatment of Sexual Disorders)

Surprisingly, the first established indication for CPA was suppression of drive in sexually deviant behaviour. CPA was introduced on the market in 1973 exclusively for this indication.
Why were we surprised? Until the mid sixties it was firmly believed that the higher a particular species stood on the evolutionary ladder, the less the libido of the male individual was dependent on androgens. This means it should be possible to inhibit the libido of the male rat with an antiandrogen to a greater extent than that of the human male. However, the opposite proved to be the case. CPA was unable or only partly able to inhibit libido and potency in the usual laboratory animals such as rats, mice, guinea-pigs and hamsters [for review see 18], whereas it has been shown to be highly effective in some other species and in humans [33-38].
Male sexuality is reduced or inhibited in the order libido - erection - orgasm. The maximum effect is attained between the 20th and 25th day of treatment.
Because spermatogenesis is an androgen-dependent process too, CPA inhibits maturation division and, when given in extremely high doses, also earlier steps of germ cell maturation (see Fig. 6).

The testicular changes are fully reversible as has been shown in patients (precocious puberty, hypersexuality) treated for 6 to 7 years continuously with high doses.
It should be mentioned that, in contrast to CPA, pure antiandrogens do not affect spermatogenesis or fertility, or only to a limited extent at the start of treatment.

Effect of CPA on Onset of Puberty and Bone Maturation (Precocious Puberty)

The rational basis for the usefulness of CPA in symptomatic treatment of precocious puberty was established in rat experiments.
If CPA is given to juvenile rats daily, starting before puberty, then the onset of puberty can be delayed for as long as desired. In this case we measured both sexual activity and fertility. Normal male rats become fully fertile in about 2 months. The capacity for insemination and fertility run closely parallel. Puberty did not occur in the group of animals that received CPA. Thirty to 40 days after cessation of treatment the animals showed the onset of puberty and became fertile [39].
It was also shown in growing male rats that CPA delays both skeletal maturation and longitudinal growth (Fig. 7) [40].

Effect of CPA on Skin and Skin Appendages

In regard to disorders of the skin, the most important effect of CPA is that on sebaceous gland function and terminal hair growth. It has been demonstrated in numerous studies (animals and humans) that sebaceous gland function is androgen dependent. It is also known that increased sebaceous gland function is of causal significance to the development of acne and seborrhoea. Figure 8 shows an example of inhibition of sebaceous gland function in mice.
CPA inhibits sebocyte proliferation as autoradiographic studies with H^3-thymidine have shown. Thymidine is incorporated in dividing cells only.
The inhibitory effect of CPA on sebaceous gland function has been confirmed in men - initially by measurements of sebum secretion in men under treatment for hypersexuality [41] and subsequently in healthy volunteers [42]. In

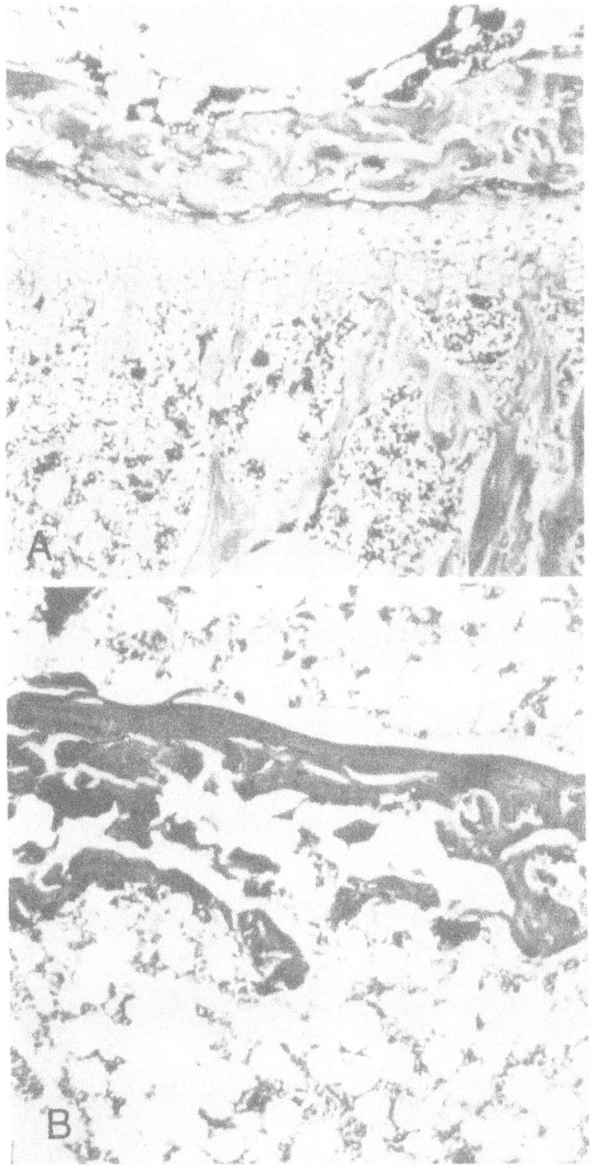

Fig. 7. Metatarsal bones of 80-day-old male rats
A Treated from day 28-80 with 6.0 mg/kg/day testosterone propionate plus 18.0 mg/kg/day cyproterone acetate s.c. (the epiphyseal space is still open, the cartilage is well maintained)
B Treated from day 28-80 with 6.0 mg/kg/day testosterone propionate s.c. (the epiphyseal space is closed)
Magnification: x 64. Staining: Haematoxylin Eosin

this study, 100 mg CPA were given orally every day and the sebum secretion rate was found to decrease by about 60% within 20 days.
Growth of terminal hair is inhibited by CPA. Symptoms of androgenisation (acne, seborrhoea, hirsutism, androgenic alopecia) are among the most important indications for CPA.

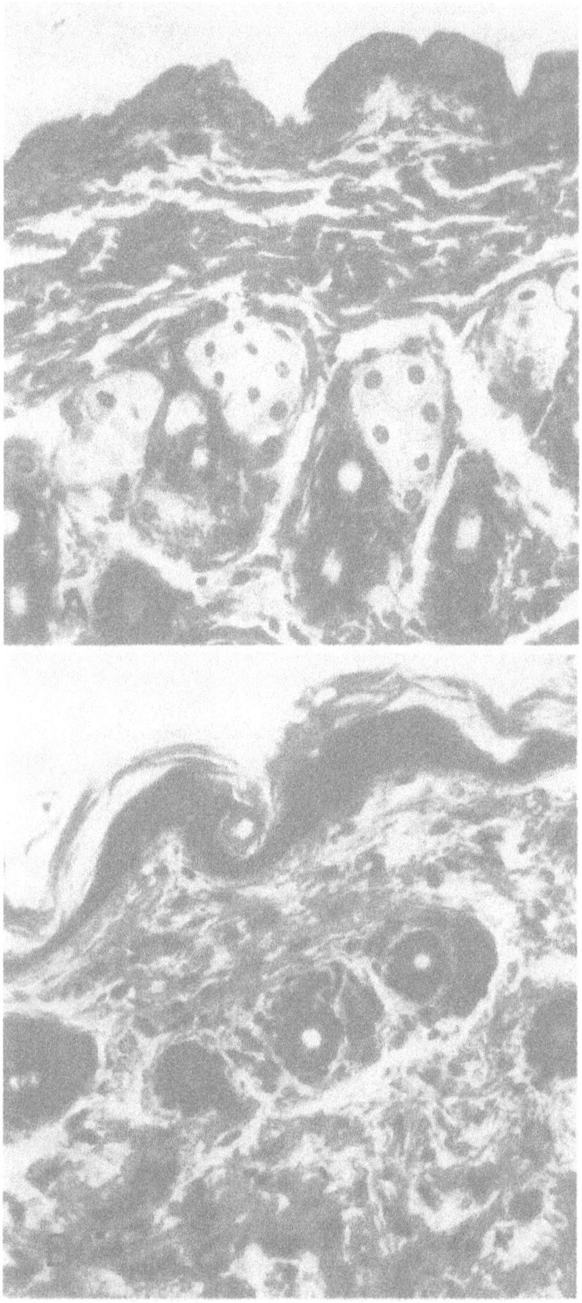

Fig. 8. Dorsal skin sections of castrated male mice after intramuscular administration of:
A 0.5 mg/48 h/animal testosterone propionate over 4 weeks
B 0.5 mg/48 h/animal testosterone propionate and 1.0 mg/48 h/animal cyproterone acetate over 4 weeks
Magnification: x 265
Staining: after Mallory

Progestational and Antigonadotrophic Activity of CPA

The progestational potency of CPA is important for its clinical use in both women and non-orchidectomised men.

CPA has been shown in classic tests to be a potent progestogen. It is one of the most effective progestogens of the group of hydroxyprogesterone derivatives [3] and has about the same range of effects as progesterone.

Like all progestogens, CPA displays therefore also antigonadotrophic properties. By this spectrum of activities, contraception is provided in women. In men, gonadotrophins and testosterone do not increase as is the case with pure antiandrogens.

Figure 9 presents for various progestogens a comparison of the oral threshold values in the Clauberg test in the rabbit with the oral transformation doses in the Kaufmann test in women. Although some of the data for the Kaufmann

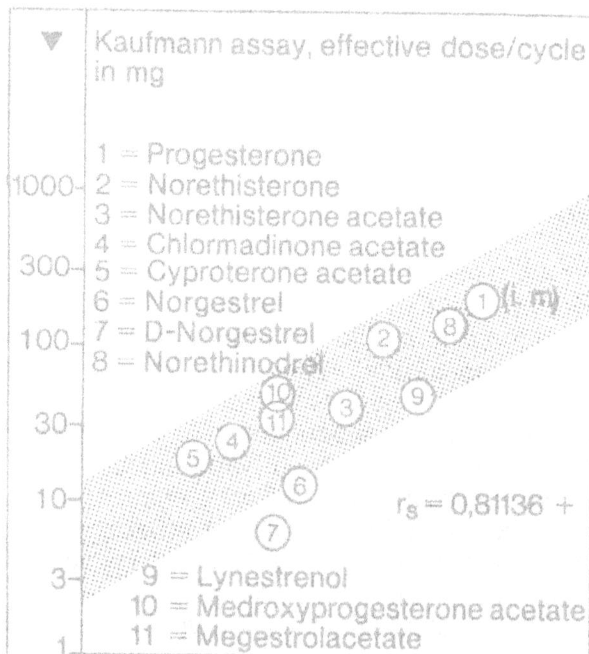

Fig. 9. Progestational potencies. Comparison of the oral transformation dose (Kaufmann test) in women with the oral threshold value (Clauberg test) in rabbits

test are most inaccurate, it can still be seen that a highly significant correlation exists between the efficacies observed in the two test models. The clinical efficacy of CPA is exceeded only by that of D-norgestrel (levonorgestrel) and norgestrel.
The anti-ovulatory effectiveness of various progestogens in women and in rats is shown in Figure 10.
The oral effective dose of CPA is about 1 mg/ day in women.

Other Endocrine Activities

Glucocorticoid-like Properties of CPA

CPA and some chemically related steroids have glucocorticoid-like properties in animals. For example, the weights of the adrenals and thymus decrease in rats and other species of laboratory animals. The adrenal atrophy is due to reduced secretion of adrenocorticotrophic hormone (ACTH) and results in reduced synthesis and secretion of glucocorticoids. For example, corticosterone levels fall in the rat and hydrocortisone in the guinea-pig. On the other hand, CPA has no anti-inflammatory properties (granuloma pouch test) and is also ineffective in the eosinophil test. Thus CPA and similar antiandrogens display only some of the typical effects of glucocorticoids. No sign of secondary adrenal insufficiency has been seen in any study.
In clinical use, glucocorticoid effects become manifest only during high-dose (more than 80-100 mg/m^2 body area) CPA therapy in children with precocious puberty. These children fail to display signs of secondary adrenal insufficiency [for review see 14,43].

Androgen-like (Agonistic) Activities of CPA

Based on rather non-specific tests for androgenicity it was claimed that CPA displays certain agonistic properties [44]. However, no evidence has been forthcoming in either rats, mice or dogs, that CPA might also have androgenic properties - at least not in the classic tests for androgenicity.

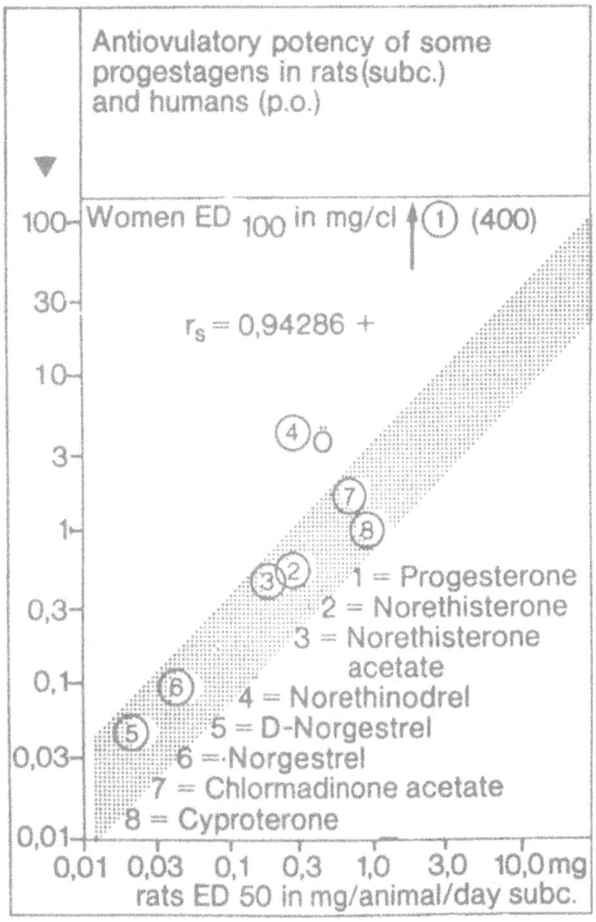

Fig. 10. Antiovulatory efficacy of various progestins. Comparison of the oral ovulation-inhibiting dose in women with subcutaneous doses in rats

In castrated rats, dosages up to 10 mg per animal per day did not lead to any increases in the weight of the prostate.
Furthermore, studies on the effect of CPA in dogs showed that it was comparable with that of surgical castration. A complete loss of secretory activity also occurs in the Huggins fistula dog after administration of CPA at a daily dosage of 10 mg over 14 days [45].
The proliferative activity of the prostate was also studied by means of H^3-labelled thymidine incorporation in the prostate [46]. The rate of incorporation of thymidine, i.e., the proliferation, in castrated animals can be substantially increased by replacement with androgens. This effect is completely abrogated by simultaneous administration of CPA. The rate of incorporation of tritium-labelled thymidine is exactly the same as that in untreated castrated controls. If CPA had any androgenic properties, then the values would lie somewhere between those of the un-

treated controls and those of the animals treated with testosterone propionate.
Clinical data available from all indications do not reveal any agonistic activity of CPA.

A Retrospective View

It has been a long and by no means always straight road from the discovery of the first antiandrogen showing clinical promise to the development of commercial preparations which are now used in urology (prostatic carcinoma), dermatology and gynaecology (acne, seborrhoea, hirsutism, alopecia), paediatrics (precocious puberty) and psychiatry (suppression of drive in sexually deviant behaviour). For the first time, some of these diseases could be treated appropriately or at least very much better than previously. One of the main problems had been that no standard existed against which we could measure this antiandrogen. Now that standard is CPA.
The development of adequate pharmacological models often proved to be difficult and time consuming. Pharmacokinetic studies were very hard to carry out because of the lack of suitable methods at that time. Problems were encountered as regards dose-finding. No one was able to predict the dosage at which CPA would have to be administered in the individual indications. Complicated dose-finding studies were therefore required.
This was also unknown territory for our colleagues in clinical research. At first, no one had any idea as to which test parameters should be used for the clinical investigation of this preparation in the different indications. How, for example, does one measure sexuality objectively? What parameters are suitable for checking the results of therapy in hirsutism?
It is interesting that CPA is still the only antiandrogen which is also used to treat non life-threatening diseases or conditions such as symptoms of androgenisation in women. Since very recently it is also used as an antiandrogenic/progestational compound in a preparation for hormone replacement therapy in postmenopausal women.
The good tolerance and low incidence of side-effects in all indications have been proven in more than 20 years of clinical experience.

REFERENCES

1 Dorfman RI: Anti-androgenic substances. In: Dorfmann RI (ed) Methods in Hormone Research. Academic Press, New York, London 1962, vol II, pp 315-323

2 Dorfman RI: Biological activity of antiandrogens. Br J Derm 1970 (82 Suppl 6):3-8

3 Wiechert R and Neumann F: Gestagene Wirksamkeit von 1-Methyl- und 1,2-Methylen-Steroiden. Arzneimittelforschung 1965 (15):244-246

4 Neumann F and Hamada F: Intrauterine Feminisierung männlicher Ratten-feten durch das stark gestagen wirksame 6-chlor-6-1.2-methylen-17-hydroxyprogesteronacetat. 10. Symp Dtsch Ges Endokrinol, Springer Verlag, Berlin, Göttingen, Heidelberg 1964

5 Hamada H, Neumann F and Junkmann K: Intrauterine antimaskuline Beeinflussung von Rattenfeten durch ein stark gestagen wirksames Steroid. Acta Endocrinol 1963 (44):380-388

6 Jensen EV: Remembrance: Gregory Pincus - Catalyst for early receptor studies. Endocrinology 1992 (131):1581-1582

7 Jensen EV and Jacobson HI: Basic guides to the mechanism of estrogen action. Recent Progr Horm Res 1962 (18):387

8 Fang and Liao S: Antagonistic action of antiandrogens on the formation of a specific dihydrotestosterone-receptor protein complex in rat ventral prostate. Mol Pharmacol 1969 (5):428-431

9 Becker H, Düsterberg B and Klosterhalfen H: Bioavailability of cyproterone acetate after oral and intramuscular application in men. Urol Int 1980 (35): 381

10 Gerhards E, Gutsche H and Riemann J: Biodynamik von Cyproteronacetat nach oraler Verabreichung beim Menschen. Arzneimittelforschung 1973 (13): 1550

11 Bhargawa AS, Seeger A and Günzel P: Isolation and identification of 15-ß-hydroxy cyproterone acetate in dog, monkey and man. Steroids 1977 (30):407

12 Speck U, Jentsch D, Kühne G, Schulze PE and Wendt H: Bioverfügbarkeit und Pharmakokinetik von Cyproteronacetat-14C nach Applikation als 50-mg-Tablette. Arzneimittelforschung 1976 (26):1717

13 Neumann F, von Berswordt-Wallrabe R, Elger W, Steinbeck H, Hahn JD and Kramer M: Aspects of androgen-dependent events as studied by antiandrogens. Recent Prog Horm Res 1970 (26):337-410

14 Neumann F: Pharmacology and clinical uses of cyproterone acetate. In: Furr BJA and Wakeling A (eds) Pharmacology and Clinical Uses of Inhibitors of Hormone Secretion and Action. Baillière Tindall, London, Philadelphia, Toronto, Mexico City, Sydney, Tokyo, Hong Kong 1987 pp 132-159

15 Neumann F and Töpert M: Pharmacology of antiandrogens. J Steroid Biochem 1986 (25 5B):885-895

16 Neumann F and Töpert M: Antiandrogens: Chemistry, pharmacology and experimental basis with special reference to the effect on the skin and its appendages. In: Orfanos CE and Happle R (eds) Hair and Hair Diseases. Springer Verlag, New York, Berlin, Heidelberg 1986 pp 791-826

17 Schleusener A, Albring M and Neumann F: Pharmacology of old and new antiandrogens. In: Jeffcoate SL (ed) Androgens and Ant-Androgen Therapy. John Wiley & Sons, Chichester, New York, Brisbane, Toronto, Singapore 1982 pp 71-93

18 Neumann F and Steinbeck H: Antiandrogens. In: Eichler O, Farah A, Herken H and Welch AD (eds) Handbook of Experimental Pharmacology. Springer Verlag, Berlin, Heidelberg, New York 1974 Vol XXXV/2 pp 235-484

19 Neumann F: The antiandrogen cyproterone acetate: Discovery, chemistry, basic pharmacology, clinical use and tool in basic research. Clin Exp Endocrinol 1994 (102 suppl):1-32

20 Neumann F, Steinbeck H and Hahn JD: Hormones and brain differentiation. In: Martini L, Motta M, Fraschini F (eds) The Hypothalamus. Academic Press, New York, London 1970 pp 569-603

21 Neumann F, Elger W and Steinbeck H: Antiandrogens and reproductive development. Philos Trans R Soc Lond B 1970 (259):179-184

22 Neumann F and Elger W: Sexual differentiation: Studies with antiandrogens. In: Serio M, Motta M, Zanisi M and Martini L (eds) Sexual Differentiation: Basic and Clinical Aspects. Raven Press, New York 1984 pp 191-208

23 Neumann F and Jacobi GH: Antiandrogens in tumour therapy. In: Furr BJA (ed) Clinics in Oncology. WB Saunders Co Ltd, London, Philadelphia 1982 pp 41-64

24 Tunn U, Senge TH, Schenck B and Neumann F: Effects of cyproterone acetate on experimentally induced canine prostatic hyperplasia. A morphological and histochemical study. Urol Int 1980 (35): 125-140

25 Tunn U, Senge TH, Schenck B and Neumann F: Biochemical and histological studies on prostates in castrated dogs after treatment with androstanediol, oestradiol and cyproterone acetate. Acta Endocrinol 1979 (91):373-384

26 Neumann F, Habenicht UF and Schacher A: Antiandrogens and target cell response - different in vivo effects of cyproterone acetate, flutamide and cyproterone. In: McKerns KW, Aakvaag A and Hanssen V (eds) Regulation of Target Cell Responsiveness. Plenum Press, New York 1984 vol II pp 489-527

27 Furr BJA: The case for pure antiandrogens. In: Furr BJA and Denis L (eds) Clinical Oncology. Baillière Tindall, London, Philadelphia, Sydney, Tokyo, Toronto 1988 pp 581-590

28 Habenicht UF, Witthaus E and Neumann F: Antiandrogens and LH-RH agonists endocrinology in the initial phase of their use. Aktuel Urol 1986 (17):10-16

29 Svensson M, Varenhorst E and Kagedal B: Initial administration of cyproterone acetate to prevent the rise of testosterone concentration during treatment with an LHRH agonist in prostatic cancer. Anticancer Res 1986 (6):379

30 Radlmaier A, Bormacher K and Neumann F: Hitzewallungen bei Endokrintherapie des Prostatakarzinoms: Modellvorstellung zu ihrer Genese. Aktuel Urol 1989 (20):143-147

31 Krämer P, Andrzejak-Nolten N, Kalischnigg and Neumann F: Prevention of hot flushes with CPA in the hormonal treatment of prostatic cancer - Results of placebo-controlled double-blind trial. In: Murphy G, Khoury S, Shatelain S and Denis L (eds) Proceedings IIIrd International Symposium on Recent Advances in Urological Cancer - Diagnosis and Treatment, Paris, June 1992. Scientific Communication Intern Ltd, Jersey 1933 pp 111-115

32 Horn HJ: Administration of antiandrogens in hypersexuality and sexual deviations. In: Eichler O, Farah A, Herken H and Welch AD (eds) Androgens II and Antiandrogens. Springer Verlag, Berlin 1974 pp 543-562

33 Neumann F and Schenck B: Antiandrogens: Basic concepts and clinical trials. In: Cunningham GR, Schill WB and Hafez ESE (eds) Regulation of Male Fertility. Martinus Nijhoff Publishers, The Hague, Boston, London 1980 pp 93-104

34 Ott F and Hoffet H: Beeinflussung von Libido, Potenz und Hodenfunktion durch Antiandrogene. Schweiz Med Wochenschr 1968 (98):1812-1815

35 Laschet U and Laschet L: Psychopharmacotherapy of sex offenders with cyproterone acetate. Pharmakopsychiatr Neuropsychopharmakol 1971 (4):99-104

36 Laschet U and Laschet L: Eine neue Möglichkeit der medikamentösen Behandlung dissozialer Jugendlicher. In: Hoffmann W and Katein W (eds) Jugend-Dissozialität. Neckar-Verlag, Villingen 1971 pp 114-117

37 Raspé G (ed) Schering Symposium über Sexualdeviationen und ihre medikamentöse Behandlung. Life Science Monographs 2. Pergamon Press, Vieweg, Oxford, Edinburgh, New York, Toronto, Sydney, Braunschweig 1972

38 Mothes C, Lehnert J, Samimi F and Ufer J: Klinische Prüfung von Cyproteronacetat (Androcur) bei Sexualdeviationen - Gesamtauswertung. Medizinische Mitteilungen (Schering AG) 1973 (2):26-39

39 Steinbeck H and Neumann F: Effect of cyproterone acetate on puberty. J Reprod Fertil 1971 (26):59-63

40 Hertel P, Kramer M and Neumann F: Einfluß eines Antiandrogens (Cyproteronacetat) auf Knochenwachstum und Knochenreifung männlicher Ratten. Arzneimittelforschung 1969 (19):1777-1790

41 Burton JL, Laschet U and Shuster S: Reduction of sebum excretion in man by the antiandrogen, cyproterone acetate. Br J Dermatol 1973 (89):487-490

42 Wendt H and Hümmelinck R: The effect of cyproterone acetate on some endocrinological parameters. In: Hammerstein J, Lachnit-Fixson U, Neumann F, Plewig G (eds) Androgenization in Women - Acne, Seborrhoea, Androgenetic Alopecia and Hirsutism. Excerpta Medica, Amsterdam, Oxford, Princeton 1980 pp 259-265

43 Girard J, Helge H, and v. Mühlendahl KE: Treatment of idiopathic precocious puberty with cyproterone acetate. Horm Res (Basel) 1978 (9):301-312

44 Poyet P and Labrie F: Comparison of the antiandrogenic/androgenic activities of flutamide, cyproterone acetate and megestrol acetate. Mol Cell Endocrinol 1985 (42):283-288

45 Bridge RW and Scott WW: A new antiandrogen, SH-714. Invest Urol 1964 (2):99

46 Sugimura Y, Cunha GR and Bigsby RM: Androgenic induction of DNA synthesis in prostatic glands induced in the urothelium of testicular feminized (Tfm/Y) mice. Prostate 1986 (9):217-225

Cyproterone Acetate - Results of Clinical Trials and Indications for Use in Human Prostate Cancer

Fritz H. Schröder

Department of Urology, Erasmus University and Academic Hospital, P.O. Box 1738, 3000 DR Rotterdam, The Netherlands

Cyproterone acetate (CPA) was first applied clinically in the management of prostate cancer by Scott and Schirmer [1]. The results of this initial experience were reported during the year 1966. Since then, cyproterone acetate has been studied in many prospective studies as monotherapy and in combination with other treatment regimens. The intent of this chapter is to summarise the results of such studies and to arrive at concluding recommendations for the clinical use of this drug.

Mechanism of Action and Pharmacokinetics

Cyproterone acetate is a steroidal antiandrogen that combines the capacity of blocking androgens at the target cell with antigonadotrophic properties; the latter are due to its gestagenic mode of action. CPA at standard dosages is completely resorbed in the intestine. Its elimination half-life after oral administration of 100 mg is 4.3 days. The pharmacokinetics, dose determination, effects in animals and animal models and *in vitro* as well as other aspects of the mechanism of action have recently been reviewed by Schröder et al. [2]. Some of the biological effects of CPA in comparison with non-steroidal, so-called "pure" antiandrogens in intact males are reviewed in Table 1. CPA leads to a decrease in testosterone (T), 5-α dihydrotestosterone (DHT), oestradiol (E2) and luteinising hormone (LH) in plasma. It also decreases hypothalamic catecholamines, which stimulate the release of LHRH but are also involved in temperature regulation. CPA in this way interferes with hot flushes. While CPA decreases or eliminates libido and potency, pure antiandrogens, due to the associated rise in plasma testosterone, do not. Gynaecomastia is commonly associated with pure antiandrogens but rarely seen with CPA.
A fairly complete review of the mechanism of action and the biological and pharmacological properties of CPA has recently been provided by Barradell and Faulds [3]. The present report will be limited to clinical aspects.

Table 1. Biological effects of CPA and "pure" antiandrogens in intact males

		CPA	Pure Anti-androgens
Plasma	T	decrease	increase
	DHT	decrease	increase
	E2	decrease	increase
	LH	decrease	increase
Hypothalamic catecholamines		decrease	?
Leydig cells		atrophy	hypertrophy
Prostate size, BPH		decrease	decrease
PC		decrease	decrease
Gynaecomastia		slight increase	pronounced increase
Libido		decrease	intact
Potency		decrease	intact

Table 2. Phase II and non-randomised comparative trials of cyproterone acetate (CPA) in prostate cancer

Author	No. pts.	Other treatment	Follow-up
Scott & Schirmer [1]	10	---	unknown
Geller [4]	11	---	unknown
Smith [5]	28	DES	unknown
Bracci [6]	236	Orchidectomy	7 years
Giuliani [7]	144	Orchidectomy	5 years
Varenhorst [8]	15	---	2 months
Isurugi [9]	19	---	3 months
Klosterhalfen [10]	28	Orchidectomy + radiotherapy	5 years
Tunn [11]	39	---	5 years
Maier [12]	70	Orchidectomy	----

Uncontrolled Clinical Studies of CPA in Prostate Cancer

Table 2 gives a list of phase II and non-randomised comparative trials as well as trials using CPA in combination with other treatment regimens. This list includes most of the available studies. Most authors describe clinically relevant effects of CPA on metastatic deposits. CPA is also reported to be associated with a volume decrease of the primary tumour, which often facilitates micturition. While in some of the studies long follow-up periods are available, comparison is not attempted; often the organisation of the studies is such that comparison is not possible with respect to the major endpoints of interest: time to progression, death of metastatic disease and overall survival.
The recommended dose of cyproterone acetate as monotherapy is 200 to 300 mg given in 3 dosages of two 50 mg tablets per day. It is remarkable that many of the studies cited used less than the recommended dose, i.e., amounts varying between 100 mg and 300 mg/day. Such variations are likely to have an impact on the outcome of the various protocols.

Phase III Randomised Trials of CPA as Monotherapy

Three major studies have been performed to compare cyproterone acetate at recommended regular dosages to standard forms of endocrine treatment, such as oestradiol and DES 3 mg. All these studies date back to the time when the effectiveness of CPA in the treatment of prostate cancer was established. The trials and their results are summarised in Table 3.
Most of the earlier randomised studies of prostate cancer included locally advanced and metastatic disease. This is true for the studies

Table 3. Phase III randomised trials of CPA monotherapy

Author	No. pts.	Comparison with CPA	Results
Jacobi [12,13]	95	Oestradiol undecylate	Fewer side effects with CPA
Pavone [14]	75	MPA, DES 3mg/day	Progression and survival better for CPA and DES Fewer cardiovascular side effects for CPA
Moffat [16]	60	Goserelin, DES 3 mg	Poorer median survival with CPA (?)

reported by Jacobi et al. [12] and also for EORTC protocol 30761 coordinated by Pavone-Macaluso [14]. Both of these studies did not find a difference in progression and survival rates between cyproterone acetate treated patients and those treated with oestradiol undecylate or DES 3 mg. Neumann and Jacobi [13], however, concluded that CPA has significantly fewer side-effects than oestradiol undecylate. Their findings mainly considered oedema and gynaecomastia. A more complete evaluation of side-effects was carried out by Pavone-Macaluso et al. [14] and De Voogt et al. [15]. These studies firmly established that cyproterone acetate has significantly fewer cardiovascular side-effects than diethylstilboestrol 3 mg/day. Both studies found a higher local response rate compared with response of distant lesions. The study by Moffat [16], which unfortunately recruited only 60 patients to the CPA arm, attempted a comparison with goserelin depot monotherapy of 3.6 mg every 28 days. Moffat found a shorter median survival time in patients receiving 300 mg of CPA/day. However, the number of patients is probably inadequate to prove this difference.

Treatment results with DES 3 mg had been previously reported by Byar and Corle [17] in an evaluation of the VACURG studies; they found survival rates identical to those obtained with castration. The same was shown by EORTC protocol 30805 with 1 mg of DES/day [21] for progression and survival rates. Castration has been considered the "gold standard" of endocrine treatment in the past and at present it is uncertain whether it could be replaced by a new "gold standard", which might be total androgen blockade. Since CPA has the same effectiveness as DES 3 mg/day, CPA in monotherapy may be considered as standard endocrine treatment.

CPA in Total Androgen Blockade Regimens

Total androgen blockade consists in the exclusion or elimination of testicular androgens together with the elimination or blockade of adrenal androgens as the initial treatment of prostate cancer. In two different prospective randomised studies, total androgen blockade by a combination of either an LHRH analogue or castration and the pure antiandrogen flutamide has been shown to significantly prolong time to progression and overall survival [18,19]. This effect may be limited to patients with favourable prognostic factors, as is pointed out in both publications. Other doubts about total androgen blockade and its possible role as "gold standard" have been expressed [20].

Two major studies have been conducted to evaluate the possible effectiveness of CPA in total androgen blockade regimens, EORTC protocols 30805 and 30843. Again, this list is incomplete, other studies, however, do not add any different points of view (Table 4) .

EORTC study 30805, reported by Robinson and Hetherington [21], compared a regimen that incompletely suppresses plasma testosterone (DES 1 mg/day) to castration as standard treatment and to castration plus cyproterone acetate 50 mg/3 times a day. Progression and survival were the endpoints of the study, which also evaluated side-effects. A total of 350 patients were entered into this protocol. All had metastatic disease at entry. No differences in time to progression or overall survival were observed.

Protocol 30843 was set up as a 3-arm study. This protocol also recruited only patients with metastatic disease. A total of 367 patients were randomised to orchidectomy as standard treatment versus the LHRH agonist buserelin plus cyproterone acetate during the first two weeks of treatment or buserelin plus cyproterone acetate 150 mg/day given continuously. No differences in the major endpoints, time to progression and duration of survival, were seen between the 3 treatment arms.

Table 4. Phase III randomised trials of CPA in combination with castration or an LHRH analogue

Author	No.pts.	Comparison with CPA	Results
Robinson [21] (EORTC 30805)	112	DES 1 mg Castration	No difference in progression and survival
De Voogt [22] (EORTC 30843)	100	Castration, LHRH + CPA for 2 wks	No difference in progression and survival

Dalesio [23] has presented an overview of all trials where total androgen blockade regimens were used, including those with CPA. Meta-analysis of the original data confirmed the results of the two randomised studies just discussed and did not show a difference in favour of total androgen blockade utilising CPA.

CPA has, however, been shown to be effective in suppressing the biochemical and clinical exacerbation (flare phenomenon) which is seen during the initial phase of LHRH agonist treatment. Klijn [24] showed that when cyproterone acetate treatment is initiated at the same time as the LHRH agonist, the initial surge in plasma testosterone cannot be suppressed. The associated surge in prostatic acid phosphatase, however, was suppressed in patients who were treated with the LHRH agonist buserelin combined with 3 times 50 mg/day of CPA. Boccon-Gibod [25] showed that when the same regimen was applied 1 week prior to the initiation of LHRH analogue treatment, also the rise in plasma testosterone could be suppressed. Therefore, in situations where the flare phenomenon could be associated with clinical symptoms, the use of CPA can be recommended in the initial phase of treatment, starting either 1 week before or at the same time as LHRH administration.

Treatment of Hot Flushes

Eaton and McGuire [26] were the first to describe effective treatment of orchidectomy-induced hot flushes by cyproterone acetate. Twelve patients were entered into their trial. The patients received CPA 100 mg/3 times daily for 3 weeks or placebo for 3 weeks. A significant decrease in the daily number of hot flushes was seen. Radlmayer et al. [27] offered an explanation for this therapeutic effect. At the level of the hypothalamus, sex steroid hormones stimulate the release of opioid peptides, which serve as inhibitory factors for hypothalamic adrenergic activity. The adrenergic substances, the catecholamines adrenaline and noradrenaline, serve as stimulatory transmitters for LHRH secretion. In particular noradrenaline also has an important thermo-regulatory effect. Hot flushes can be explained by accumulation and release of noradrenaline, which subsequently leads to a rise in peripheral body temperature. This effect is prevented by CPA, which by its gestagenic action is able to release the hypothalamic inhibitory factors and prevent the accumulation of noradrenaline.

Side-Effects of Cyproterone Acetate

The use of cyproterone acetate in the treatment of prostate cancer leads to loss of libido and potency. Exceptions have been described, however: men who remain potent and sexually active under CPA treatment are seen from time to time in clinical practice.

Gynaecomastia is not a significant complication of CPA treatment. Hot flushes due to LHRH agonist therapy can be prevented by cyproterone acetate [22].

Table 5. Cardiovascular side-effects

	No history of CV disease		History of CV disease				
	Side-effects		Side-effects		Total side-effects		
Treatment	**no**	**yes**	**no**	**yes**	**no**	**yes**	**Total**
CPA	37	3 (8%)	12	5 (29%)	49	8 (14%) *	57
MPA	28	10 (26%)	21	5 (19%)	49	15 (23%) **	64
DES	25	12 (32%)	11	10 (48%)	36	22 (38%) ***	58
Total	90	25 (22%)	44	20 (32%)	134	45 (25%)	179

* 4 CV deaths ** 1 CV death *** 2 CV deaths

Reproduced with permission from [29]

Cardiovascular side-effects have been attributed to the use of CPA. The possibility of cardiovascular side-effects is in fact mentioned in the product description. The available information in the literature, however, does not seem to point in this direction; on the contrary, all comparative studies show that cardiovascular symptoms occur less frequently with CPA than with oestrogens and are equivalent in CPA-treated patients and control groups (castration, LHRH treatment). Wallentin and Varenhorst [28] showed that plasma lipoproteins (HDL and LDL) and plasma testosterone are reduced after 2 and 8 weeks of treatment. The most extensive study of cardiovascular side-effects has been carried out by the EORTC-GU Group and has been reported by De Voogt et al. [15,29] (Tables 5 and 6). The data of these prospective randomised studies clearly show that in patients with and without a previous history of cardiovascular disease, CPA was associated with a considerably lower percentage of cardiovascular side-effects. The cardiovascular side-effects observed consisted mainly of ischaemic cardiopathy, thromboembolic disease and fluid retention. However, the number of cardiovascular deaths was highest in the CPA-treated group of 57 patients recruited in EORTC protocol 30761. Unfortunately, no study is available that allows a placebo comparison.

Table 6. Type of cardiovascular complications

Prot. 30761	DES	MPA	CPA
Ischaemic cardiopathy	10.5	6	3.5
Thromboembolic diseases	10.5	6	3.5
Fluid retention	17	6	7
Not specified	0	2	0
Total	38	20	14

Figures represent percent values
Reproduced with permission from [29]

Table 7 summarises the cardiovascular disease related deaths in all EORTC studies with CPA and reports on the cardiovascular death rates in EORTC protocol 30853, which compared castration to depot LHRH agonist goserelin plus flutamide. The regimens of protocol 30853 have never been described as being associated with an increased incidence of cardiovascular death. Castration arms are also present in studies 30805 and 30843. The last column indicates the percent of cardiovascular deaths among patients who died in the different treatment arms. It is evident that no excessive rate of cardiovascular deaths can be attributed to the use of cyproterone acetate in these studies.

Table 7. Cardiovascular disease-related deaths in EORTC studies

EORTC 30761, De Voogt et al. [15]			
CPA	N=57	CV deaths 4/57	(7.0%)
MPA	N=64	CV deaths 1/64	(1.6%)
DES 3 mg	N=58	CV deaths 2/58	(3.5%)
EORTC 30805, Robinson et al. [21]			
Castration	N=90	CV deaths 4/90	(4.4%)
Castration + CPA	N=86	CV deaths 1/86	(1.2%)
DES	N=86	CV deaths 4/86	(4.7%)
EORTC 30843, De Voogt et al. [22]			
Castration	N=104	CV deaths 8/104	(7.7%)
Buserelin + CPA 2 weeks	N= 98	CV deaths 6/98	(6.1%)
Buserelin + CPA	N=100	CV deaths 3/100	(3.0%)
EORTC 30853, Denis et al. [19]			
Castration	N=163	CV deaths 11/163	(6.8%)
Goserelin + Flutamide	N=164	CV deaths 12/164	(7.3%)

Hepatic toxicity has been described in association with the use of CPA. This was usually but not always reversible.

Conclusions

In conclusion, cyproterone acetate given orally at standard dosages has proved to be effective in the treatment of prostate cancer. Its effectiveness has been shown both in response of the primary tumour and in response of metastatic disease. In one randomised study cyproterone acetate was demonstrated to be superior to low-dose medroxyprogesterone acetate. It has also been shown to be equally effective as 3 mg DES/day. In these studies CPA was associated with significantly fewer cardiovascular side-effects than other treatments. The rate of cardiovascular deaths is probably comparable to that in trial populations treated with other forms of endocrine management. In this regard CPA treatment can be considered equivalent to treatment by castration.

The use of CPA has not shown any advantages in terms of progression rates, prostate cancer death rates or overall survival in total androgen blockade trials, where a comparison was made between castration, an LHRH agonist and LHRH plus CPA during the first two weeks of treatment. CPA, however, has been shown to efficiently counteract the biochemical and clinical flare associated with the initial surge of plasma testosterone under LHRH agonist treatment. Cyproterone acetate is capable of preventing hot flushes induced by castration or LHRH agonists. It is effective in decreasing the side-effect of gynaecomastia which may accompany LHRH agonist treatment.

The side-effect profile of CPA is, therefore, quite acceptable. CPA can be recommended in the treatment of prostate cancer for the indications mentioned above, as an alternative to castration.

REFERENCES

1 Scott WW and Schirmer HK: A new oral progestational steroid effective in treating prostatic cancer. Trans Am Assoc Genito-Urin Surg 1966 (58):54-62
2 Schröder FH: Cyproterone acetate - Mechanism of action and clinical effectiveness in prostate cancer treatment. Cancer 1993 (72):3810-3815
3 Barradell LB and Faulds D: Cyproterone, a review of its pharmacology and therapeutic efficacy in prostate cancer. Drugs & Aging 1994 (5):59-80
4 Geller J, Vazakas G, Fruchtman B et al: The effect of cyproterone acetate on advanced carcinoma of the prostate. Surg Gynecol Obstet 1968 (127):748-758
5 Smith RB, Walsh PC, Goodwin WE: Cyproterone acetate in the treatment of advanced carcinoma of the prostate. J Urol 1973 (110):106-108
6 Bracci U: Antiandrogens in the treatment of prostatic cancer. Eur Urol 1979 (5):303-306
7 Giuliani L, Pescatore D, Giberti C, Martorana G, Natta G: Treatment of advanced prostatic carcinoma with cyproterone acetate and orchiectomy - 5 year follow-up. Eur Urol 1980 (6):145-148
8 Varenhorst E: Metabolic Changes During Drug Treatment in Carcinoma of the Prostate. Linköping University Medical Dissertation 1980 p103
9 Isurugi K, Fukutani K, Ishida H, Hosoi Y: Endocrine effects of cyproterone acetate in patients with prostatic cancer. J Urol 1980 (123):180-183
10 Klosterhalfen H (ed) Endocrine Management of Prostate Cancer. De Gruyter, Berlin 1988
11 Tunn UW: Antiandrogen Therapie des fortgeschrittenen Prostata Karzinoms. Springer Verlag, Berlin1987 pp 113-124
12 Jacobi GH, Altwein JE, Kurth KH, Basting R, Hohenfellner R: Treatment of advanced prostatic cancer with parenteral cyproterone acetate: a phase III randomised trial. Br J Urol 1980 (52):208-215
13 Neumann F and Jacobi GH: Antiandrogens in tumour therapy. Clin Oncol 1982 (1):41-64
14 Pavone-Macaluso M, de Voogt HJ, Viggiano G, Barasolo E, Lardennois B, de Pauw M, Sylvester R: Comparison of diethylstilbestrol, cyproterone acetate and medroxyprogesterone acetate in the treatment of advanced prostatic cancer: final analysis of a randomized phase III trial of the European Organization for Research on Treatment of Cancer Urological Group. J Urol 1986 (136):624-631
15 de Voogt HJ, Smith PH, Pavone-Macaluso M, de Pauw M, Suciu S and Members of the European Organization for Research on Treatment of Cancer Urological Group: Cardiovascular side effects of diethylstilbestrol, cyproterone acetate, medroxyprogesterone acetate and estramustine phosphate used for the treatment of advanced prostatic cancer: results from European Organization for Research on Treatment of Cancer Trials 30761 and 30762. J Urol 1986 (135):303-307
16 Moffat LEF: Comparison of Zoladex, diethylstilbestrol and cyproterone acetate treatment in advanced prostate cancer. Eur Urol 1990 (18 suppl3):26-27
17 Byar DP and Corle DK: Hormone therapy for prostate cancer: results of the Veterans Administration Cooperative Urological Research Group Studies. NCI Monographs 1988 (7):165-170
18 Crawford ED, Eisenberger MA, McLeod DG, Spaulding JT, Benson R, Dorr FA, Blumenstein BA, Davis MA, Goodman PJ: A controlled trial of leuprolide with and without flutamide in prostatic carcinoma. N Engl J Med 1989 (321):419-429
19 Denis LJ, Carneiro de Moura JL, Bono A, Sylvester R, Whelan P, Newling D, de Pauw M: Goserelin acetate and flutamide versus bilateral orchiectomy: a phase III EORTC trial (30853). Urol 1993 (42):119-130
20 Schröder FH: Endocrine therapy: where do we stand and where are we going? Cancer Surv 1991 (11 - Prostate Cancer):177-194
21 Robinson MRG and Hetherington J: The EORTC studies: Is there an optimal endocrine management for M1 prostatic cancer? World J Urol 1986 (4):171-175
22 de Voogt HJ, Klijn GM, Studer U, Schröder F, Sylvester R, de Pauw M, Members of the EORTC-GU Group: Orchidectomy versus buserelin in combination with cyproterone acetate for 2 weeks or continuously, in the treatment of metastatic prostatic cancer. Preliminary results of EORTC trial 30843. J Steroid Biochem Molec Biol 1990 (37):965-969
23 Dalesio O: Oral communication 1994
24 Klijn JGM, de Voogt HJ, Schröder FH, de Jong FH: Combined treatment with buserelin and cyproterone acetate in metastatic prostatic carcinoma. Lancet 1985 (ii):493
25 Boccon-Gibod L, Laudat MH, Dugue MA, Steg A: Cyproterone acetate lead-in prevents initial rise of serum testosterone induced by LHRH analogs in the treatment of metastatic carcinoma of the prostate. Eur Urol 1986 (12):400-402
26 Eaton AC and McGuire N: Cyproterone acetate in treatment of post-orchidectomy hot flushes. Lancet 1983 (ii):1336-1337
27 Radlmaier A, Bormacher K, Neumann F: Hot flushes: mechanism and prevention. In: Treatment of Prostatic Cancer - Facts and Controversies. EORTC Genitourinary Group Monograph 1990 (8):131-140
28 Wallentin L and Varenhorst E: Plasma lipoproteins during treatment with cyproterone acetate in men with prostatic carcinoma. J Clin Endocrinol Metab 1980 (51):1118-1122
29 de Voogt HJ: Cyproterone acetate as monotherapy in prospective randomized trials. In: Treatment of Prostatic Cancer - Facts and Controversies. EORTC Genitourinary Group Monograph 1990 (8):85-91

Biological Properties of Flutamide

Rudolph O. Neri

Schering-Plough Research Institute, 2015 Galloping Hill Road, Kenilworth, New Jersey 07033, U.S.A.

Great interest has been generated in the past few years to uncover agents which inhibit the actions of androgens. This interest is based on the inference that such agents would be therapeutically useful in human benign prostatic hyperplasia and adenocarcinoma, hirsutism, and acne.

Several compounds have been shown to be more or less effective in antagonising various actions of androgens. Generally, tests have employed the ability of these compounds to either inhibit the effect of androgens on chick comb growth or the androgen-induced hypertrophy of the secondary sex structures of immature, orchidectomised rodents. Knuth et al. [1] and Neri et al. [2] reported that cyproterone acetate (1,2α-methylene-6-chloro, 4,6 pregnadiene-17α, ol-3, 20 dione-17-acetate), a potent progestational agent, possessed strong antiandrogenic activity in rats.

In addition to the steroidal antiandrogen, several non-steroidal antiandrogens have been reported. Dorfman [3] showed that dihydroisosteviol inhibited the action of testosterone on the chick comb but not on the seminal vesicles or ventral prostate of the androgen-stimulated castrate rat.

Methylcholanthrene, benzpyrene and 5-fluorouracil were also shown to inhibit the action of testosterone on the chick comb [3]. Randall and Selitto [4] reported that a perhydrophenanthrene derivative (2-acetyl-7-oxo-1, 2, 3, 4, 4a, 4b, 5, 6, 7, 9, 10, 10α-dodecahydrophenanthrene) inhibited the action of testosterone on both the chick comb and the accessory sex glands of the castrate rat. This compound was not oestrogenic but was slightly androgenic and inhibited pituitary gonadotrophin secretion in parabiotic rats.

It is evident that many of these compounds are not effective in all the tested species and/or also exhibit other hormonal actions that may negate their usefulness as antiandrogens in human therapeutics. Our efforts at Schering were directed towards the discovery of an antiandrogen with minimal or no endocrinological effects and with a wide spectrum of species sensitivity.

In this report, we describe a potent non-steroid antiandrogen (trifluoro-2-methyl-4'-nitro-m-propionotoluidide). Typical endocrinological bioassays indicate it to be devoid of other hormonal activity. The only other effect of note of this compound is its ability to elicit methaemoglobin formation in cats and to a markedly lesser degree or not at all in other species.

Intact Rat Study

Male rats (Charles River CD strain), 21-28 days old and weighing approximately 60 g, were used to assess the ability of flutamide to inhibit endogenous androgens (Table 1). The compound was suspended in an aqueous medium (0.9% NaCl, 0.5% carboxymethylcellulose, 0.4% polysorbate 80, 0.9% benzyl alcohol or CMC) and administered orally by stomach tube each day for 3 weeks. Twenty-four hours following the last drug treatment, seminal vesicles, ventral prostates, adrenals and testes were removed, freed of extraneous tissues, weighed, and placed in 10% buffered formalin for histological evaluation. Flutamide significantly reduced ventral prostate weights at doses of 1 to 25 mg/kg in intact rats. Seminal vesicle weights were significantly reduced at 10 mg/kg. Of the other organs examined (adrenals, testes) no significant weight changes were observed. Histological examination of the various tissues revealed no significant

Table 1. Effect of orally administered flutamide on organ weights in immature male rats (5 rats per group)

Treatment	Daily dose (mg/kg)	Initial body weight (g ± SE)	Final body weight (mg ± SE)	Seminal vesicles (mg ± SE)	Ventral prostate (mg ± SE)	Adrenals (mg ± SE)	Testes (mg ± SE)
Control	--	67 ± 1	213 ± 3	118.6 ± 15.1	205.1 ± 14.2	35.6 ± 1.6	2250 ± 56
Flutamide	25	62 ± 3	202 ± 5	30.5 ± 3.3**	93.1 ± 5.7**	38.7 ± 2.5	2210 ± 92
Flutamide	10	64 ± 2	195 ± 6	57.8 ± 5.5**	129.7 ± 11.3*	38.4 ± 1.3	2290 ± 11
Flutamide	5	61 ± 2	206 ± 9	81.9 ± 14.1	138.2 ± 8.4*	40.3 ± 2.3	2145 ± 31
Flutamide	1	66 ± 1	198 ± 11	91.4 ± 12.6	133.4 ± 17.5*	41.1 ± 0.9	2196 ± 66

* Significantly different from controls $p < 0.05$
** Significantly different from controls $p < 0.01$

changes compared to controls, with the exception of the seminal vesicles and ventral prostates. At doses that produced significant weight reductions for these two tissues, epithelial cells were flattened with no evidence of secretory material within the lumina of the glands. By comparison, cells lining the vesicles of control animals were tall columnar and exhibited secretory granules along with secretory material in the lumen.

Orchidectomised Rat Study

Male rats (about 60 g) were bilaterally orchidectomised, and 1 day following surgery flutamide (suspended in CMC) was given orally concomitantly with testosterone propionate (given subcutaneously in sesame oil) daily for 7 days. Twenty-four hours following the last injection, seminal vesicles and ventral prostates were removed and weighed.

Table 2. Antiandrogenic activity of flutamide in orchidectomised immature rats - 7-day study (Agonist: testosterone propionate)

Treatment	Daily dose	Number of rats	Seminal vesicles (mg ± SE)	Ventral prostate (mg ± SE)
Control (castrate)		9	7.3 ± 0.5**	12.6 ± 0.7**
Testosterone propionate (T.P.) (1)	1 10 µg	9	14.9 ± 1.0	47.2 ± 4.8
T.P. and Flutamide (2)	10 µg and 25 mg/kg	5	9.1 ± 0.3**	18.7 ± 1.3**
T.P. and Flutamide	10 µg and 10 mg/kg	5	9.2 ± 1.0**	18.2 ± 1.3**
T.P. and Flutamide	10 µg and 5 mg/kg	5	9.8 ± 0.3**	19.6 ± 1.1**
T.P. and Flutamide	10 µg and 1 mg/kg	4	10.3 ± 0.7**	36.1 ± 5.5
Flutamide	25 mg/kg	5	6.7 ± 0.9**	13.2 ± 0.9**

(1) Administered subcutaneously in sesame oil (2) Administered orally in CMC
** Significantly different from testosterone propionate-treated rats $p < 0.01$

Results in Table 2 show that flutamide effectively blocked the testosterone propionate-induced hypertrophy of the seminal vesicles and ventral prostate. The seminal vesicle weights were also depressed at 1 mg/kg. Flutamide (25 mg/kg) given alone had no effect on either the seminal vesicle or prostate weights, indicating the lack of any androgenic properties for flutamide. When either testosterone, androstenedione or dihydrotestosterone was administered with flutamide, ventral prostate and seminal vesicle weights were similarly reduced.

Studies on Rat Fetal Endocrinology

Fetal Anogenital Measurements

This study was undertaken to reveal the antiandrogenic (feminising) and possible masculinising properties of flutamide. Adult, female Charles River CD rats showing a pro-oestrus or oestrus vaginal smear were caged with males (2 females with 1 male). Twenty-four hours following cohabitation, vaginal smears were taken again and the presence of sperm was determined as an indication of successful mating and for the assignment of this day as day 1 of pregnancy. Gravid rats were given flutamide (25 mg/kg or 50 mg/kg) orally from the 16th to the 19th day of gestation. On the 21st day, the fetuses were removed by caesarotomy, and the sex of each fetus was determined by macroscopic caliper measurements of the anogenital distance with subsequent histological examination of the gonads. Each fetus was bisected transversely, and the posterior half placed in Bouin's solution. After 14 days' fixation, the fetuses were embedded in paraffin, serially sectioned (10 μ) along the sagittal median plane and stained with methylene blue. The anogenital distance (ventral margin of the anus to the external orifice or the urethra) was measured with a dissecting microscope fitted with an ocular micrometer. Five measurements were made on each fetus. The results shown in Table 3 indicate that flutamide reduced the anogenital distance of male fetuses at doses of 5-50 mg/kg. Apparently, flutamide competes with the androgens of the fetal testes for the androgen receptors of target tissues necessary for the differentiation of the male genitalia and development proceeds towards the female structure.

Table 3. Effect of flutamide on the anogenital distance in rat fetuses, caesarian delivered on day 21. Pregnant rats treated orally from days 16-19

Treatment	Daily dose (mg/kg)	Number of fetuses	Sex of fetuses	Mean anogenital distance (mm ± SE)
Control	---	4	male	3.04 ± 0.04
		8	female	1.18 ± 0.01
Flutamide	50	4	male	1.24 ± 0.03**
		5	female	1.13 ± 0.04
Flutamide	25	7	male	1.24 ± 0.03**
		5	female	1.07 ± 0.01
Flutamide	10	4	male	1.57 ± 0.20**
		3	female	1.12 ± 0.15
Flutamide	5	5	male	2.11 ± 0.04**
		3	female	1.02 ± 0.08
Flutamide	1	5	male	2.89 ± 0.14
		3	female	1.04 ± 0.24

* Significantly different from controls $p < 0.05$
** Significantly different from controls $p < 0.01$

Effect on Early Development

When flutamide was administered to gravid rats from day 16-19, parturition occurred normally and spontaneously on day 22. At autopsy, at 30 and 60 days of age, prostates were either absent or markedly atrophied. Seminal vesicle weights were also reduced compared to appropriate controls. The external genitalia of the male rats, however, revealed distinct anomalies. The penis was hypospadiac and resembled a clitoris. Immediately below the ventral prepuce, a vaginal tract was present. Epithelial cells and leukocytes were present in this tract. After the administration of oestradiol-17B, cornified squamous epithelial cells were found, a typical positive oestrus response in female rats following oestrogen stimulation. The majority of male rats had one descended testis contained within an incompletely formed scrotum. The contralateral testis was usually found embedded within subcutaneous tissue or within the peritoneal cavity. Because of these female-like structures, these male rats were considered to be "feminised".

Effects on Benign Prostatic Hyperplasia in Dogs

Three aged (6-10 years) beagle dogs (10-15 kg) with naturally occurring prostatic hyperplasia (BPH) (as determined initially by rectal palpation of the prostate) were selected for this study. The exact age of the dogs was not known but was inferred from physical examination (lens opacity, dental wear and discolouration). Under pentobarbital:pentothal (3:2), the prostate glands were exposed by an abdominal midline incision and caliper measurement (length, width and dorsoventral depth) of the organs and wedge biopsies were taken before and after treatment. In all cases, the drug was administered orally in gelatin capsules daily for 1 year, beginning 7-10 days following laparotomy. A complete blood study was performed prior to treatment and each week during treatment. This included quantitative analyses for methaemoglobin. For histological examination, each prostate wedge was cross-sectioned at 4 levels and examined using the following criteria: 1) epithelia - the height of 10 cells from various areas of the prostate were measured, and 2) stroma - sections were stained with a trichrome stain. A subjective estimate of relative amounts of smooth muscle and fibrous tissue in the stroma was made and expressed as a ratio since diffuse distribution of the stroma negated precise quantitation. The degree of reaction was rated on a graduated scale of 0 (no demonstrable enzyme) to 3 (dense staining). At biopsy and autopsy, sections of testes also were taken for histological examination by light microscopy.

The effects of flutamide on canine prostatic hyperplasia are summarised in Table 4. The dimensions of the prostate (length, width and dorso-ventral depth) expressed as cm^3 were reduced at 5 mg/kg, the minimum effective dose. This dose was selected following a dose-ranging study from 1-50 mg/kg. These reductions in prostate volume occurred at 3, 6 and 12 months. Epithelial cell height was also drastically reduced after 1 year of treatment. Methaemoglobinaemia was not significantly altered from baseline.

In one dog, daily treatment for 1 year with flutamide was suspended and the dog was autopsied 8 weeks later. Without flutamide for 8 weeks, the prostate volume and epithelial cell heights reverted to the hyperplastic state.

Antiprostate Studies in Baboon

Flutamide, diethylstilboestrol and Estracyt ® (oestradiol nitrogen mustard) were examined for their antiprostatic effect [5]. According to the authors, the prostate of this sub-human primate resembles that of man in some respects and was investigated as a possible model for the study of chemotherapeutic agents for cancer of the prostate in humans. Flutamide (5 mg/kg) was injected intramuscularly 3 times a week for 4 weeks. Following treatment, all drugs were shown to produce a definite decrease in the weight of the prostate. The mean prostate weight of the 3 baboons treated with flutamide was 3.44 g, a decrease of 66% from the mean control prostate weight of 10.18 g. Estracyt ® and diethylstilboestrol diphosphate (3 baboons/each) given intravenously in doses of 5 mg/kg reduced the weight of the prostate 32% and 42%, respectively.

Table 4. Effects of flutamide on prostatic hyperplasia and methaemoglobin formation in dogs

Dog number	Treatment [a]	Prostate volume (cm^3)	Epithelial cell height ($\mu \pm SE$)	Methaemoglobin (percent) [d]
	Initial biopsy	26.2	31.8 ± 2.6	0.8
1	3 months	12.5	—	0.3
	6 months	10.6	—	1.5
	Autopsy (1 yr)	5.3	1.6 ± 0.2*	0.5
	Initial biopsy	48.2	38.0 ± 2.8	0.1
2	3 months [b]	35.7	—	0.1
	6 months [b]	22.7	—	0.3
	Autopsy (1 yr) [b]	10.1	25.2 ± 1.9*	0.3
	Initial biopsy	28.8	33.4 ± 3.8	0.2
	3 months	14.9	—	0.5
3	6 months	15.6	—	0.5
	1 year biopsy [c]	12.5	4.8 ± 0.3*	0.7
	Autopsy (60 wks)	38.3	29.2 ± 3.4	0.6

a 5 mg/kg p.o. daily for 1 year
b Cystic prostate
c Daily treatment stopped after 1 year. Dog autopsied 8 weeks later
d In terms of haemoglobin
* Significantly different from initial biopsy $p < 0.01$

Effect of Flutamide and Leuprolide on the Growth of Dunning R-3327 Prostatic Adenocarcinoma in Copenhagen Rats

It has been reported that the Dunning R-3327 rat prostatic carcinoma mimics many of the characteristics of the human disease [6] and has been used to study the question of tumour growth and androgen dependence. Kung et al. [7] carried out studies to determine whether combining flutamide with leuprolide elicited a greater reduction in tumour size than either modality alone. Once the rats had palpable tumours (128-142 days after implantation into the flanks), they were orchidectomised and adrenalectomised and placed on 0.9% normal saline in their drinking water. Flutamide (15 mg/kg p.o.) and leuprolide (25 µg s.c.) were administered daily for 4 weeks. Castrated controls produced a dramatic decrease (93%) in tumour size followed by flutamide (76%) and leuprolide (44%). When flutamide was combined with leuprolide, the decrease in tumour size was 89%. When therapy was stopped, the tumours resumed their growth.

Mechanism of Action

Peets et al. [8] studied the effect of flutamide on ^3H-dihydrotestosterone uptake and metabolism in rat ventral prostates and compared it to the steroidal antiandrogen, cyproterone acetate. The results indicated that both flutamide and cyproterone acetate administered p.o. at 15 mg/kg/4 days markedly inhibited ^3H testosterone and ^3H-dihydrotestosterone uptake and retention by prostate and prostate nuclei when labelled androgen was given 3 hours following the last dose of drug. However, when added to rat ventral prostate *in vitro*, flutamide's effect of labelled androgen uptake was attenuated, suggesting that flutamide might achieve its results, at least in part, through an active metabolite.

Methaemoglobin Formation

Because flutamide is an anilide, its potential for methaemoglobin production was investigated in several animal species. Results corroborated the reported species sensitivity to acetanilide in animals.

Flutamide (100 mg/kg) administered orally to 5 cats for approximately 2 weeks, caused a progressive increase in serum methaemoglobin levels, to a maximum of almost 30% after 1 week. When administration of flutamide was discontinued, methaemoglobin levels returned rapidly to control values.

In a comparative study, flutamide (50 mg/kg) in carboxymethylcellulose suspension was administered by gavage to guinea pigs, rats, cats, dogs, squirrel monkeys and rhesus monkeys for 2 weeks. In the 3 cats tested, the mean concentration of methaemoglobin rose to 31% in 48 hours, and remained between 20% and 30% during treatment. Because of emesis, none of the cats could be treated longer than 10 days. The 4 dogs, however, had only sporadic changes in methaemoglobin concentrations. Mean values were approximately 14% at 7 hours, but these decreased to normal at 24 hours and remained there for the rest of the treatment period.

In guinea pig, rat, squirrel monkey and rhesus monkey, methaemoglobinaemia did not occur at any time during the experiment.

Other Pharmacological Activities

Effects on Spermatogenesis

Flutamide (25 mg/kg) administered orally to rats once daily for 30 days, did not affect spermatogenesis and did not alter the morphology of Leydig cells. The secretory activity of the epididymis either remained unaffected or was stimulated. There was a significant decrease in seminal vesicle and ventral prostate weight and in fructose content of coagulating glands. There was no change in pituitary gland weight.

Effects on Serum Cholesterol

Immature rats receiving flutamide 50 mg/kg/day orally for 3 weeks had serum cholesterol levels (70 mg%) not significantly different from control levels (70 mg%).

Effects on the Cardiovascular System

Intravenous administration of flutamide to anaesthetised dogs caused the following:

a. at 1 mg/kg - slight (mean 13%) reduction in heart rate;
b. at 5 mg/kg - slight (17%) increase in blood pressure in 1 of 3 dogs;
c. at 20 mg/kg - transient increase in blood pressure (mean 33%), in heart rate (mean 41%) and contractile force/beat (mean 44% in 2 of 3 dogs). One dog (chloralose anaesthesia) showed transient nodal rhythm. There were no other electrocardiographic changes at any doses.

In another experiment, 3 unanaesthetised dogs each received one dose of flutamide; one dog received 20 mg, the other two 100 mg. Direct and electrocardiographic monitoring of the dogs for 5 to 6 hours after drug administration did not indicate any toxic effects on the heart.

The effect of flutamide on thrombus formation was studied in male and female rats. Occlusive arterial thrombosis was achieved by insertion of a polyethylene cannula into the abdominal aorta. Administration of depo-testosterone cypionate increased thrombus formation resulting in a 4-fold increase in the mortality rate in male and female rats. When flutamide (50 mg/kg) was injected subcutaneously once daily for 2 weeks together with depo-testosterone cypionate (10 mg/kg) subcutaneously twice a week, a decrease in thrombus formation was observed and the mortality rate was reduced by approximately 50% as compared to the group receiving androgen alone.

Metabolism

Single oral doses of flutamide ranging from 50 mg/kg to 100 mg/kg given to dogs, rats and cats resulted in peak plasma concentrations of the drug and its metabolites in about 7 hours in the cats and 4 to 6 hours in the other species. Chronic administration of these daily dose levels resulted in drug accumulation in the dog but not in the other species.

In the monkey, the estimated half-life of an intravenous dose was 45 to 90 minutes. Oral studies in the monkey suggested that flutamide was rapidly absorbed from the gastrointestinal tract and rapidly and extensively metabolised.

Other studies conducted in various species, including man, corroborated those findings and demonstrated that hydroxyflutamide was the major metabolite [9]. The suggestion that hydroxyflutamide was responsible for most of flutamide antiandrogenic properties was substantiated by several *in vitro* studies [10-13].

Studies in Man - Phase I

Flutamide, administered orally at daily doses ranging from 10 mg to 1500 mg, given in single or multiple doses, was evaluated in healthy volunteers and cancer patients. Three phase I clinical trials delineated the tolerance and pharmacodynamics of flutamide in volunteers.
The safety and efficacy of flutamide were evaluated in controlled studies, including two double-blind studies and one open study.

Studies in Normal Healthy Volunteers

Rising single-dose tolerance study

The safety of and tolerance to flutamide were evaluated in a single-dose, double-blind, placebo-controlled, parallel-design study conducted in normal male volunteers. Forty-two healthy male subjects, aged 21 to 38 years, were enrolled in the study. Medical history, physical examination and laboratory tests were completed before each volunteer was randomly assigned to one of 6 treatment groups, each composed of 5 flutamide and 2 placebo subjects. Each subject received only one single dose of flutamide (10, 50, 100, 150, 300, 600 mg) or placebo.
Vital signs were recorded at 0, 6, 24 and 72 hours following drug administration. Complete blood counts and blood chemistries were determined on day 0, and 24 and 72 hours after drug administration. Methaemoglobin determinations were performed at 0, 6-8, 24, and 72 hours after drug administration.
Analysis of the laboratory tests, including liver and kidney functions, as well as the function of the cardiovascular and haematopoietic systems, revealed no flutamide-induced toxicity. Methaemoglobin levels remained within normal limits. Subjective symptoms such as decreased appetite, sleepiness, headache, urinary hesitancy, insomnia, tranquillity, dry mouth and nausea were occasionally reported in both flutamide and placebo groups, and were not deemed to be drug-related.
It was concluded that flutamide was a safe and well-tolerated drug when given in rising single doses (10 mg to 600 mg) to healthy male volunteers.

Three-week subacute tolerance in normal adult volunteers

This was a 2-phase, double-blind tolerance study in which normal healthy male volunteers received flutamide in multiple daily doses for 21 days.
Twenty-four male volunteers, 21 to 37 years old, were enrolled in the study. Fifteen subjects were enrolled in the first phase of the study and randomly assigned to one of 3 treatment groups. Six volunteers received 75 mg of flutamide TID, 6 received 150 mg TID, and 3 received placebo. When no signs of intolerance were observed, 9 additional subjects were entered in the second phase of the study and randomly assigned in a 2 to 1 ratio to receive 250 mg of flutamide TID or placebo.
Tolerance to flutamide was monitored by recording vital signs, ECGs and analysing laboratory tests (blood chemistries, formed elements of blood, organ functions, hormone levels, sperm count and morphology). Subjective adverse experiences were also documented throughout the trial.
Few subjects reported symptoms. All reported symptoms were mild. There was no consistent pattern of progression of symptoms. Side-effects were neither dose-related nor drug-related since similar symptoms, such as increased appetite, headache, thirst, nausea, tiredness, dizziness and constipation were reported in both flutamide and placebo groups. Mean values for total white blood cell counts were within the normal range, as were plasma testosterone, LH, FSH, and cortisol levels. Sperm count and sperm morphology were not adversely affected.
It was concluded that flutamide given TID orally to normal male volunteers at total daily doses of 225 mg, 450 mg and 750 mg for 21 days, was well tolerated and had no adverse effects on blood chemistries and sperm counts and morphology.

Pharmacodynamic effects of flutamide in normal male volunteers

A 6-week, double-blind, placebo-controlled study was designed to evaluate the pharmacodynamic effects of flutamide (500 mg TID or 125 mg TID) by monitoring routine blood and urine chemistries, plasma hormone levels, clotting factors and sperm counts, morphology and motility in healthy volunteers.
Twenty-six healthy young adult male volunteers, 21 to 23 years old, were enrolled in the study. Five withdrew before completion of the study for reasons unrelated to the administration of flutamide. Seven of the subjects received oral doses of flutamide 500 mg TID, 7 received 125 mg TID, and 7 received placebo TID. The dosage regimens were given for 6 weeks. Blood, urine and seminal fluid samples were collected at set intervals during the study. Possible adverse experiences were recorded weekly.
Routine blood and urine analyses revealed no significant changes during or after drug administration. Clotting factors VII, IX and XII and methaemoglobin levels were not elevated beyond normal levels. Plasma levels of FSH, LH, prolactin, dihydrotestosterone, PBI and thyroxine were not significantly different from placebo during or after treatment.
The only major complaint reported by any volunteer was nipple tenderness and/or development of firm, tender subareolar nodules or small tender nodules in the periphery of the breast and the existence of colostrum. These complaints were reported by 5 of 7 subjects on the high dose and 2 of 7 on the low dose of flutamide. One other volunteer on the high dose developed unilateral nodules without nipple tenderness during the sixth week of treatment. Colostrum could be expressed from the nipples of 6 of these 8 subjects.
A trend showing dose-related increases in plasma testosterone during treatment was noted.
Plasma oestradiol levels showed a dose-related increase during drug administration. Plasma oestrone levels were higher in those subjects who developed gynaecomastia than in those who did not. In addition, those subjects who developed gynaecomastia had a higher incidence of amorphous and immature sperms in the fourth week than those who did not. Whether gynaecomastia is indirectly related to the rise in the plasma oestradiol or some metabolite of testosterone is conjectural at this point.

Acknowledgement

The author extends a grateful acknowledgement to Misses Gallagher, Garcia and Ventura for the preparation of this manuscript.

REFERENCES

1 Knuth UA, Hano R, Nieschlag E: Effect of flutamide or cyproterone acetate on pituitary and testicular hormones in normal men. J Clin Endocrinol Metab 1984 (59):963-969

2 Neri RO, Florence K, Koziol P, Van Cleave S: A biological profile of a nonsteroidal antiandrogen, SCH 13521 (4'-nitro-3'-trifluoromethylisobutyranilide). Endocrinology 1972 (91):427-437

3 Dorfman RI: The antiandrogenic activity of a phenanthrene derivative in the chick. Endocrinology 1959 (64):464-465

4 Randall LO and Selitto JJ: Antiandrogenic activity of a synthetic phenanthrene. Endocrinology 1958 (62): 693-695

5 Muntzing J, Varkarakis MJ, Yamanaka H et al: Studies of antiprostatic agents in the baboon. Proc Soc Exper Med 1974 (146):849-854

6 Dunning UF: Prostate cancer in the rat. NCI Monographs 1963 (12):351-369

7 Kung TT, Mingo G, Siegel M, Watnick A: Effect of adrenalectomy, flutamide and leuprolide on the growth of the Dunning rat, R-3327, prostatic carcinoma. The Prostate 1988 (12):357-363

8 Peets E, Henson F, Neri RO: On the mechanism of the antiandrogenic action of flutamide (alfa, alfa, alfa, trifluoro-2-methyl-4-nitro-m-propionotoluidide) in the rat. Endocrinology 1974 (94):532-540

9 Katchen B and Buxbaum S: Disposition of a new, nonsteroid antiandrogen, alpha, alpha, alpha trifluoro-2-methyl-4'-nitro-m-propionotoluidide (flutamide) in men following a single oral 200 mg dose. J Clin Endocrinol Metab 1975 (41):373-379

10 Liao S, Howell DK, Chang TM: Action of a nonsteroid antiandrogen (flutamide) on the receptor binding and nuclear retention of 5 alpha dihydrotestosterone in the rat ventral prostate. Endocrinology 1974 (94): 1205-1209

11 Mainwaring WP, Mangam FR, Feherty PA, Freidfeld M: An investigation into the antiandrogenic properties of the nonsteroid antiandrogen SCH 13521 (4 nitro 3' trifluoro-methylisobutyranilide). Molec Cell Endocrinol 1974 (1):113-128

12 Ghanadian R, Smith CB, Williams G, Chisholm GD: The effect of antiandrogens and stilbestrol on the cytosol receptor in rat prostate. Br J Urol 1977 (49): 695-700

13 Symes EK, Milroy EJG, Mainwaring WP: The nuclear uptake of androgen by human benign prostate in vitro: action of antiandrogens. J Urol 1978 (12):180-183

Combination Therapy with Flutamide: The Therapy of Choice from Early to Advanced Stages of Prostate Cancer

Fernand Labrie, André Dupont, Leonello Cusan, José-Luis Gomez, Raul Suburu and Pierre Diamond

CHUL Research Center and Laval University Medical Center, 2705 Boulevard Laurier, Quebec G1V 4G2, Canada

Among all hormone-sensitive cancers, prostate cancer is recognised as being the most sensitive. In fact, the best known characteristic of prostate cancer is its marked sensitivity to androgen deprivation: when surgical or medical castration is used [1], a procedure limited to the blockade of testicular androgens, a response of limited duration is observed in 60% to 80% of patients [2]. Such a high rate of positive responses is already quite impressive since, as will be discussed later, testicular androgens account for only 60% of total androgens in 65-year-old men, thus leaving approximately 40% of androgens free to continue to stimulate prostate cancer [3].

Following recognition of the importance of the formation of dihydrotestosterone (DHT) in the prostate [3-6], our research efforts turned towards defining the structure of the genes encoding the enzymes responsible for the intraprostatic formation of DHT. We have thus elucidated the structure of most of the cDNAs and genes encoding the enzymes responsible for the conversion of the adrenal precursor dehydroepiandrosterone (DHEA) into DHT, namely 3β-hydroxysteroid dehydrogenase/Δ^5-Δ^4 isomerase, 17β-hydroxysteroid dehydrogenase and 5α-reductase [7,8, and references therein]. These major advances provide us with the molecular biology tools required to understand the mechanisms of androgen formation and action in the human prostate and thus be in a better position to design improved therapeutic approaches. This presentation, however, is centered on the clinical data obtained with flutamide as part of combination therapy at all stages of the disease. In fact, recent data strongly suggest that combination therapy should be used not only in advanced disease, but also in combination with other approaches (prostatectomy or radiotherapy) in the early stages of prostate cancer.

Adrenal Androgens are Responsible for 40% (and not 5-10%) of Total Androgens in Men

Although castration (by orchidectomy or chemically by luteinising hormone-releasing hormone (LHRH) agonists) causes a 95% reduction in serum testosterone concentration, a much more limited effect is seen on the intraprostatic concentration of DHT, which is the only meaningful parameter of androgenic action in the prostatic tissue. In fact, after elimination of testicular androgens by medical or surgical castration, the intraprostatic concentration of DHT remains at approximately 40% of that measured in intact 65-year-old men (Fig. 1A). As another measure of the importance of adrenal androgens in adult men, the serum levels of the main metabolites of androgens - 5α-androstane-3α, 17β-diol (3α-diol), androsterone (ADT), and their glucuronidated derivatives - are only reduced by 50%-70% [9,10] following castration, thus reflecting the high level of adrenal precursor steroids converted into DHT in castrated men (Fig. 1B). Contrary to the previous, erroneous belief that the testes are responsible for 95% of total androgen production, as suggested by simple measurement of circulating serum testosterone, it is now well demonstrated that the prostatic tissue efficiently transforms the inactive adrenal steroid precursors dehydroepi-

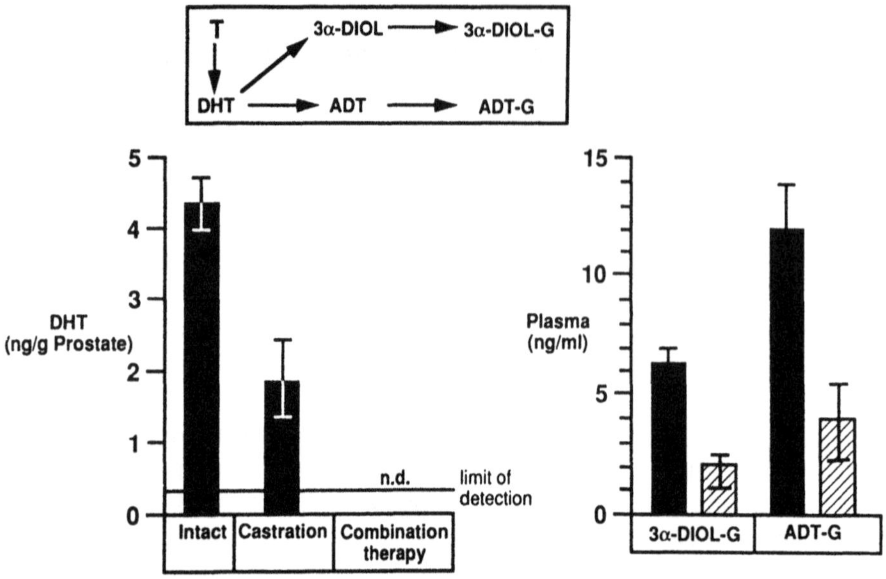

Fig 1. (A) Effect of orchidectomy or combination therapy (addition of flutamide to orchidectomy or treatment with an LHRH agonist) on the concentration of DHT in human prostatic cancer tissue. (B) Effect of castration on the serum levels of ADT and 3α-diol and their respective glucuronidated derivatives [61]

androsterone sulphate (DHEA-S), DHEA and androstenedione (Δ^4-dione) into the active androgen DHT.

Simultaneous Blockade of Androgens of Both Testicular and Adrenal Origin is the Endocrine Therapy of Choice in All Stages of Prostate Cancer

Treatment of Stage D_2 Disease

Taking into account the role of both the testes and the adrenals in androgen formation in men, combination therapy was developed to simultaneously block both sources of androgens at the start of therapy in advanced prostate cancer [3,6,11] (Fig. 2). While the testicular androgens can be blocked by orchidectomy [1] or treatment with an LHRH agonist [12], we have chosen a pure antiandrogen to block the other source of DHT, namely the access of DHT of adrenal origin to the androgen receptor in prostate cancer tissue [6,11].

Flutamide was the first antiandrogen shown to possess pure antiandrogenic properties [13]. This compound prevents binding of the androgens testosterone and DHT to the androgen receptor without exerting any detectable androgenic, oestrogenic or other hormonal and antihormonal activity [14,15]. Androgen-sensitive cancer cells, on the other hand, are well known to develop a wide range of sensitivities to androgens upon exposure to low levels of androgens [16,17]. The presence of tumour clones hypersensitive to androgens requires maximal androgen blockade or the use of a pure antiandrogen having no intrinsic androgenic activity [15].

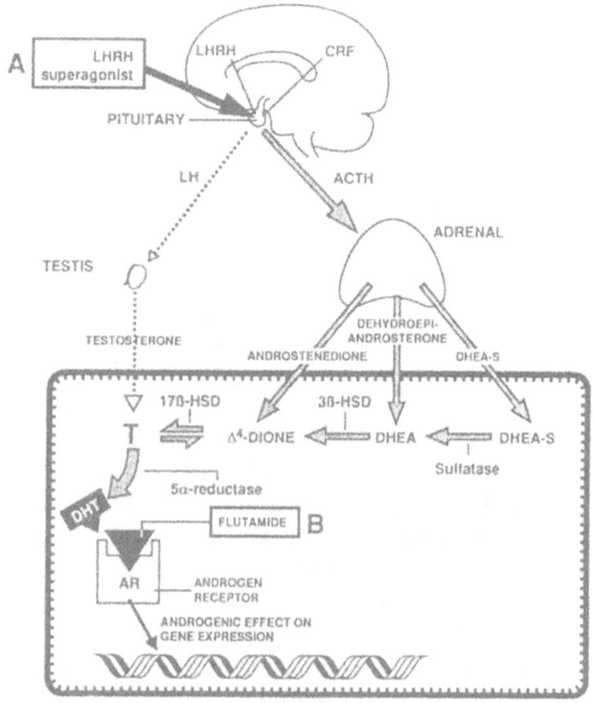

Fig. 2. Schematic representation of the effect of combination therapy with an LHRH superagonist and a pure antiandrogen (flutamide) on prostate cancer growth

Table 1. Combination therapy with flutamide and castration in stage D2 disease. Double-blind, randomised and prospective studies

	PSA or PAP normalization	Duration of response (mo)	Death due to cancer (mo)	Death from all causes (mo)
NCI Crawford et al. (602 pts) [1]	$p < 0.05$	16.9 vs 13.8 (3.1 months) $p < 0.05$		35.6 vs 28.3 (7.3 months) $p < 0.05$
EORTC (327 pts) [2]	$p < 0.05$	17.7 vs 11.3 (6.4 months) $p < 0.008$	43.9 vs 28.8 (15.1 months) $p < 0.007$	34.4 vs 27.1 (7.3 months) $p < 0.02$

The numbers in parentheses denote time in months
PSA, prostate-specific antigen; PAP, prostatic acid phosphatase; n.s., not significant
[1] flutamide and luteinising hormone-releasing hormone agonist versus LHRH agonist as control
[2] flutamide and LHRH agonist versus orchidectomy as control

The advantages of combination therapy with flutamide, first reported by our group [3,6], have been confirmed by two large-scale, double-blind and placebo-controlled randomised studies [18,19]. These pivotal studies have demonstrated the important advantages of flutamide-containing combination therapy for all objective and subjective parameters studied. Of utmost importance is the observation that the mere addition of flutamide added on average 7.3 [18] and 15.1 [19] months of life. In the EORTC 30853 study, the median time to objective progression was 85 weeks for the orchidectomy group and 133 weeks for the combination therapy group, i.e., an advantage of 48 weeks for the group of men who received flutamide ($p = 0.002$).

When all causes of death were considered, the median duration of survival was 27.1 months for orchidectomy and 34.4 months for combination therapy ($p = 0.02$). When only deaths due to malignant disease were taken into account, the group of patients who received combination therapy with flutamide had their life prolonged by 15.1 months (52%), from a median time to death of 28.8 months (orchidectomy) to 43.3 months [19] (Table 1).

The use of maximal androgen blockade at the start of therapy is well supported by the fact that patients relapsing after castration or treatment with oestrogens or LHRH agonists show a poor or no response to adrenalectomy, hypophysectomy or flutamide [3]. Moreover, a strong indication of the harmful effect of exposure of prostate cancer cells to low androgen levels by monotherapy is the recent finding that low serum testosterone levels are associated with shorter survival following androgen deprivation [20]. In fact, low serum testosterone levels before the start of endocrine therapy are associated with a poor prognosis, this variable being even more important than the extent of bone metastases [20]. All these convincing clinical data are well supported by our laboratory findings that low levels of androgens, comparable to those found after castration in men, induce the development of androgen-hypersensitive tumours, which are resistant to antihormonal therapy [17].

Such dramatic negative effects of partial androgen blockade or low androgen levels leading to shorter survival [3,11,18,19,21,22] make the use of any therapy having less androgen-blocking capacity than combination therapy including a pure antiandrogen, in association with surgical or medical castration, unethical. In fact, the participants in the Geneva meeting on prostate cancer judged that it was unacceptable to treat men suffering from prostate cancer with any treatment exerting a blockade of androgens inferior to that achieved by combination therapy [23]. The health regulatory agencies should therefore take changes in serum testosterone levels as a surrogate parameter of response when assessing the efficacy of new LHRH agonists or new formulations of these compounds, instead of using survival as the parameter of response. It is, in fact, well demonstrated that men receiving an LHRH agonist or castraction alone will lose up to 15.1 months of life [18,19].

Importance of starting treatment as soon as a diagnosis has been made

An important observation in all studies of stage D_2 prostate cancer patients who received combination therapy as initial treatment is that prostate cancer is rapidly and extremely well controlled at the level of the prostate. Moreover, when progression occurs after an initial response, the cancer reappears in the bones in approximately 98% of cases, while progression in the prostate is rare (2%). These findings clearly indicate that combination therapy is most efficient in blocking cancer growth at the level of the prostate, while the main problem of hormonal treatment is represented by tumours that have migrated and developed outside the prostatic area, usually in the bones. Such data strongly suggest that major efforts should be directed towards earlier treatment of the disease by combination therapy.

In order to further investigate the impact of early versus late treatment of metastatic prostate cancer, we stratified our cohort of stage D_2 prostate cancer patients according to the number of bone lesions. As illustrated in Figure 3, the median survival was not yet reached at 8 years in the group of patients having 1-5 bone metastases, while survival was dramatically reduced to 3.56 years when the number of bone lesions was 6-10, a difference of more than 4.4 years of life. For patients having 11-40 bone lesions, the calculated median survival was 2.36 years while it was reduced to 1.76 years for those having disseminated disease or a superscan at the start of treatment.

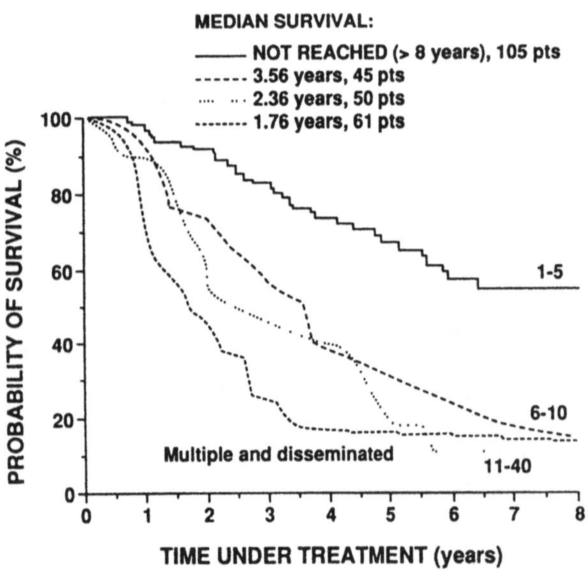

Fig. 3. Probability of survival according to the number of bone metastases, in previously untreated stage D2 prostate cancer patients who received combination therapy with flutamide and the LHRH agonist [D-Trp^6, des-Gly-NH_2^{10}] LHRH ethylamide

It is thus clear from the present data that the addition of a relatively small number of bone lesions has a major negative impact on survival. In fact, it can be seen in Figure 3 that when the number of bone metastases is larger than 5, a further increase has less and less influence on the duration of survival under combination therapy, thus clearly demonstrating the major importance of not delaying treatment once the diagnosis of metastatic prostate cancer has been made.

In agreement with these data, Crawford et al. [18] reported that patients presenting with minimal disease show a much better response to combination therapy. Recent analysis of the Intergroup NCI study has shown a survival advantage of 19.5 months for patients with minimal disease receiving a combination of leuprolide and flutamide compared to those treated with leuprolide and placebo, while the median overall survival advantage calculated for the whole group of patients was only 7.3 months following combination therapy. Similarly, in the EORTC 30853 trial, combination therapy with goserelin and flutamide in patients with a good (performance status 0-2, modest prostate-specific antigen (PSA) elevation and T category <4) or intermediate prognosis led to a markedly improved disease-free survival as well as overall survival, compared with the total group of patients [19].

Response to flutamide withdrawal

Faced with the poor results obtained in patients showing progression of the disease under any form of endocrine therapy [24-28], we have examined the possibility of an effect of withdrawal of flutamide in 40 stage D_2 prostate cancer patients who progressed after a relatively long period of positive response to treatment with the antiandrogen combined with a luteinising hormone-releasing hormone agonist or orchidectomy. A withdrawal response has already been reported with the antioestrogen tamoxifen in breast cancer patients [29,30]. Somewhat surprisingly, 30 of the 40 patients who were progressing under combination therapy showed a positive clinical response as assessed by slight modifications of the NPCP criteria [31,32].

Following withdrawal of flutamide, 1 patient (2.5%) had a complete response, 3 (7.5%) had partial responses, 26 (65%) had objective stable disease and 10 (25%) continued to progress. The average time of response after flutamide withdrawal was 14.5 months (range 3.6 to 29.9). There was no statistical correlation between the initial duration of response to combination therapy and the duration of response on withdrawal of the antiandrogen (r = 0.409).

Serum PSA levels were higher than normal (normal ≤3 μg/l) in all patients before withdrawal of flutamide. As can be seen by 6 examples shown in Figure 4, serum PSA decreased sharply after flutamide withdrawal in the responders. Following withdrawal of the antiandrogen, serum PSA returned to normal in 17 of the 30 responders (57%), while it remained above 3 μg/l in all non-responders. The decrease in serum PSA was 90% or more in 19 of the 30 responders (63%) and in only 1 of the 10 non-responders (10%). The percentage of serum PSA decrease correlates positively (r=0.578, probability level=0.0001) with the duration of response.

The low rate of complete and partial responses observed in this study is rather typical of the type of responses achieved with various approaches offered to advanced prostate cancer patients who show disease progression under endocrine therapy [3,5,24-28,33,34]. However, in our study the percentage of stable responses is higher (65%) than previously observed (11.8%) upon addition of aminoglutethimide (AG) and low-dose hydrocortisone (HC) in the same category of patients who continued to receive a luteinising hormone-releasing hormone agonist and flutamide [27]. Moreover, on addition of AG and HC, 85.7% continued to have progression compared to only 25% in the present study. Therefore, flutamide withdrawal appears to be the first therapeutic choice in patients progressing after a positive response to combination therapy.

Treatment of Stage C Disease

A considerable proportion of patients have clinical stage C disease at the time of first diagnosis [35]. The standard therapeutic approaches proposed for these patients are radiotherapy, radical prostatectomy and immediate or delayed partial androgen deprivation (orchidectomy or oestrogens) [36,37]. In a recent study we have shown that the lipoprotein profile resulting from combination therapy was more favourable than that observed following orchidectomy and especially oestrogen therapy [38,39]. In fact, oestrogen therapy induced hypertriglyceridaemia while hypercholesterolaemia as well as elevated total and LDL apolipoprotein B levels were associated with orchidectomy. Combination therapy, on the other hand, had no effect on plasma lipids and apolipoprotein B concentrations while VLDL lipoprotein apolipoprotein B decreased and LDL apolipoprotein B increased. Since combination therapy offers an advantageous serum lipid profile during long-term management of prostatic cancer patients and delayed treatment of prostate cancer permits further tumour cell dedifferentiation and the development of tumour heterogeneity [16,17,40], we have studied the effect of combined antihormonal therapy using the antiandrogen flutamide and the LHRH agonist [D-Trp[6], des-Gly-NH_2[10]]LHRH ethylamide in 115 previously untreated patients with clinical stage C prostate cancer. A comparison was made with the published results using conventional approaches.

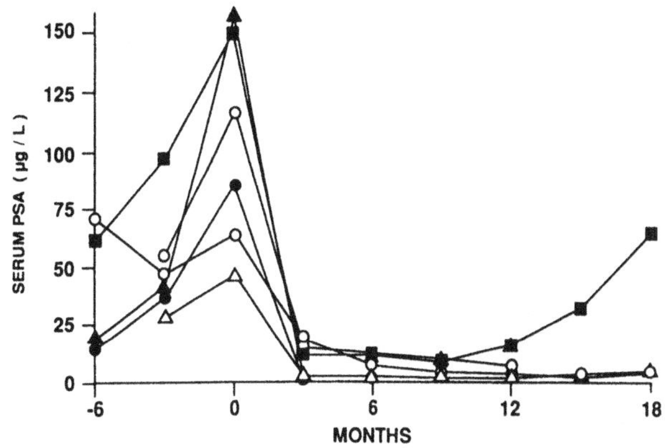

Fig. 4. Effect of discontinuation of flutamide on serum PSA concentration in stage D2 prostate cancer patients who had progression of disease under combination therapy with a luteinising hormone-releasing hormone agonist/orchidectomy associated with flutamide [44]

As shown in Table 2, all evaluable patients had a positive objective response to treatment. Moreover, after an average follow-up period of

Table 2. Best objective response achieved in 108 previously untreated stage C prostate cancer patients who received combination therapy with flutamide and the LHRH agonist [D-Trp^6, des-Gly-$NH_2{}^{10}$]LHRH ethylamide

	Median time of treatment (days)	Best objective response		
No. pts.	(limits)	Regression	Stable	Progression
108	1427 (19-3502)	95 (88%)	13 (12%)	0

1427 days or 3.9 years, 28 patients were seen to relapse. The probability of continuing response calculated according to Kaplan and Meier [41] was 98.4%, 91.2%, 85.8%, 78.2%, 74.3%, 63.5%, 60.4% and 56.4% years at 1, 2, 3, 4, 5, 6, 7 and 8 years, respectively.

The evolution of survival in the same group of patients is illustrated in Figure 5. When all causes of death were included, the calculated survival rate was 96.9 ± 1.8% (SEM), 93.4 ± 2.6%, 85.5 ± 3.9%, 82.7 ± 4.3%, 69.7 ± 5.5%, 67.7 ± 5.7%, 65.4 ± 5.9%, 51.2 ± 6.1% at 1, 2, 3, 4, 5, 6, 7 and 8 years, respectively. Twenty patients died of prostate cancer while 10 died of other causes (5 of myocardial infarct, 1 of pneumonia, 1 committed suicide, 2 died of cerebrovascular lesions, and 1 following cardiac surgery complications). It is well known from previous studies that stage C prostate cancer patients have a high risk of early progression and short survival [37,40,42,43]. The present finding of only 28 patients progressing after an average follow-up of 3.9 years is very encouraging. In fact, at 3 years the probability of a continued response is calculated at 85.8% [44].

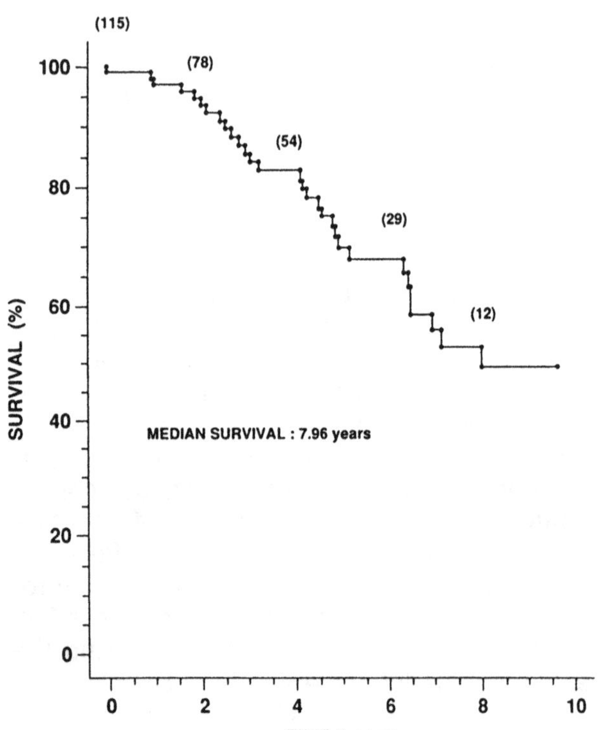

Fig. 5. Probability of survival in previously untreated patients with clinical stage C prostate cancer who received combination therapy with flutamide in association with the LHRH agonist [D-Trp^6, des-Gly-$NH_2{}^{10}$]LHRH ethylamide [44]

The present data indicate that the early administration of combination therapy using a pure antiandrogen (flutamide) in association with medical castration [D-Trp^6, des-Gly-$NH_2{}^{10}$] LHRH ethylamide to stage C prostate cancer patients has advantages over standard therapies and delayed treatment [45-47]. Although progression to stage D_2 is an early sign of treatment failure, it is of interest to compare, at this stage of our study, the survival rate observed under combination therapy with the results obtained in other studies using monotherapy. The death rate at 2 years with combination therapy is 6.6% while it is, on average, 34% (5.5-fold difference) at the same time interval following treatment with DES or Estracyt [47]. In the EORTC study, the death rates at 2 years of treatment with cyproterone acetate, DES and medroxyprogesterone acetate were 12%, 22% and 31%, respectively [46]. When the above-mentioned data are pooled (513 patients), the average death rate at 2 years is 22.2% with standard therapy as compared to only 6.6% in the present study (3.3-fold difference).

Treatment of Stage B Disease

Although it is well recognised that the only opportunity for cure of prostate cancer is treatment at an early stage, radical prostatectomy has remained relatively unpopular. The controversy in the treatment of early stage prostate cancer is mainly due to the observation that 40% to 50% of prostate cancers estimated at diagnosis as being confined to the prostate are found to be at a more advanced stage following histopathological analysis of the specimen removed at surgery, which is an indication that these patients have a high risk of recurrence. In 5 series including 1457 patients with clinical stage T_1 or T_2 carcinoma of the prostate, only 680 (47%) had tumour confined to the prostate on pathological examination [48-52]. In a study of 439 patients who had radical prostatectomy for stage T_2 disease at Johns Hopkins, only 34% of the tumours were found to be organ confined [53]. Rosen et al. [51] discovered that only 37% of 98 patients with clinical stage T_2 disease had pathological stage T_2 disease.

The importance of organ-confined disease at surgery has been well described by Frazier et al. [50]. With a mean follow-up of slightly more than 3 years, a 3.9% clinical failure rate was observed in patients having organ-confined disease at the time of radical prostatectomy, while a PSA increase was seen in 9.8% of cases. However, in specimen-confined disease, 39% had evidence of detectable clinical or PSA failure. In the group of men having positive margins at surgery, 13% had clinical evidence of failure and 68% had a detectable increase in serum PSA. Such data stress the importance of organ-confined disease at surgery.

Recent non-randomised studies have clearly indicated that preoperative or neoadjuvant combination therapy with the antiandrogen flutamide and a luteinising hormone-releasing hormone (LHRH) superagonist before radical prostatectomy [5,54-60] could decrease the incidence of cancer not confined to the surgical specimen (cancer-positive margins) at the time of surgery. As a follow-up of our initial study [58] we have conducted the first prospective and randomised clinical trial to assess the potential beneficial effects of neoadjuvant therapy with the antiandrogen flutamide and an LHRH superagonist on the incidence of cancer-positive margins at radical prostatectomy and on the histopathological stage of the cancer determined at surgery compared with clinical staging at diagnosis.

Table 3. Effect of 3-month neoadjuvant combination therapy with the antiandrogen flutamide and an LHRH agonist on positive margins at radical prostatectomy in stage B and C prostate cancer

Group	Negative margins	Positive margins	Total
Control	40 (61.5%)	25 (38.5%)	65
Combination therapy	67 (87.0%)	10 (13.0%)	77
Total	107	35	142

Chi-square test: p = 0.006

As expected, cancer-positive surgical margins were found in 38.5% (25 of 65) of control patients, whereas the incidence of positive margins was dramatically reduced to only 13.0% (10 of 77) ($p = 0.006$) in the group of patients who received the LHRH superagonist and flutamide for 3 months before radical prostatectomy (Table 3). Figure 6 shows that the decrease in cancer-positive surgical margins is of major amplitude in all stages of the disease except in stage B_0, where the number of patients in each group was only two. In fact, although positive margins were found in the surgical

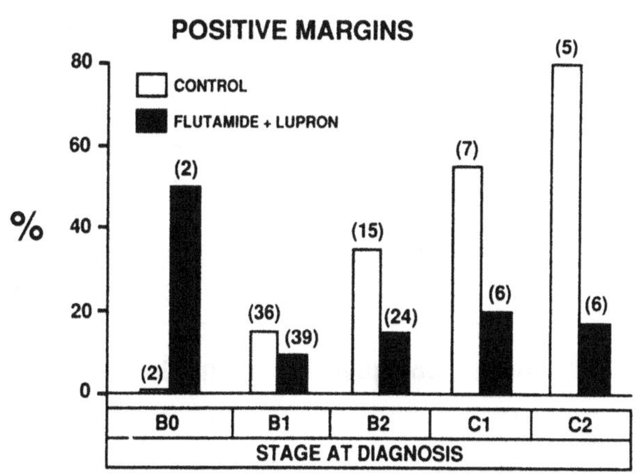

Fig. 6. Effect of 3-month neoadjuvant combination therapy with flutamide and an LHRH agonist on cancer-positive margins at radical prostatectomy in specific stages of prostate cancer determined at diagnosis. The numbers in parentheses indicate the number of patients in each group

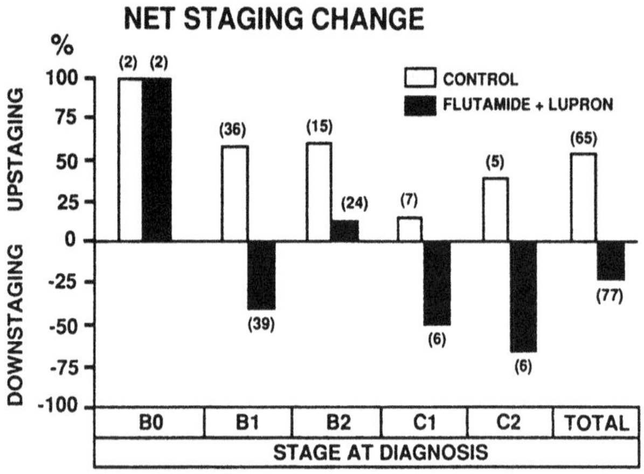

Fig. 7. Comparison of final stage at histopathological examination of the surgical specimen and clinical staging at diagnosis in men who had radical prostatectomy alone (control group) and those treated for 3 months with the combination flutamide and an LHRH agonist before radical prostatectomy. The numbers in parentheses indicate the number of patients in each group [61]

specimens in 15% of stage B_1, 35% of stage B_2, 55% of stage C_1, and 80% of stage C_2 control patients, the incidence of margins positive for cancer decreased to 9% in stage B_1, 15% in stage B_2, 20% in stage C_1 and 17% in stage C_2 patients who received combination therapy for 3 months before surgery (Wilcoxon test, $p = 0.04$).

Figure 7 shows the net effect on staging at histopathological analysis compared with initial staging at diagnosis. Net upstaging occurred in 53.8% of control patients; in contrast, 23.4% of cases were downstaged at analysis of the surgical specimen in the group of patients who had combination therapy before surgery, for a net difference of 77.2% in favour of neoadjuvant combination therapy.

It is thus of particular interest to examine more closely the effect of combination therapy at each stage (Table 4). Upstaging is particularly striking at stages B_1 and B_2 in the control group. In fact, of 36 cancers originally classified as B_1, 22 showed a more advanced stage at surgery, including 8 C_1 and 11 C_2 disease. Similarly, of 15 cancers originally classified as B_2 disease in the control group, 2 became C_1, 8 became C_2, and 1 became D_1. Of special interest is the finding that of 6 patients originally classified as having biopsy-proven clinical stage C_1 disease, 3 were downstaged to B_2 at surgery in the neoadjuvant group. Moreover, of the 6 patients having initial C_2 disease or in-

Table 4. Effect of 3-month neoadjuvant therapy with flutamide and an LHRH agonist on the final histopathological stage at surgery compared to the initial clinical stages at diagnosis

A. Control

Original Stage	No.	Final histopathological stage at surgery B_0	B_1	B_2	C_1	C_2	D_1
B_0	2	0	0	0	2	0	0
B_1	36	1	13	3	8	11	0
B_2	15	0	2	2	2	8	1
C_1	7	0	0	1	4	2	0
C_2	5	0	0	0	1	1	3

B. 3-month neoadjuvant combination therapy

Original Stage	No.	Final histopathological stage at surgery B_0	B_1	B_2	C_1	C_2	D_1
B_0	2	0	0	0	1	1	0
B_1	39	17	17	0	1	4	0
B_2	24	1	4	11	4	3	1
C_1	6	1	0	3	1	1	0
C_2	6	1	1	3	0	0	1

volvement of the seminal vesicles proven by biopsy, 5 of the 6 cancers were downstaged to stage B disease, and only one was found at surgery to be stage D_1.

It is well known that perineural space invasion is frequently associated with capsule penetration in stage B prostate carcinoma [62,63]. In fact, perineural space invasion has been reported to be responsible for capsule penetration in 50% of all cases [63]. Moreover, one study reported that prostate capsule penetration by perineural space (PNS) invasion near the apex was accompanied by positive margins in 89% of cases [63]. In the present study, 50% (18 of 36) of positive margins were associated with PNS invasion following radical prostatectomy alone; this value was reduced to 16.0% (8 of 50) in the treated group (Fig. 8). In the absence of demonstrated PNS invasion, 24% of positive margins were observed in the control group while in patients receiving neoadjuvant therapy only 10.8% were found to have cancer-positive margins.

Although the impact of neoadjuvant combination therapy on survival remains to be evaluated by long-term follow-up, it seems reasonable to expect, as has been demonstrated by Brendler and Walsh [64], that patients with organ-confined disease at surgery should have a life expectancy similar to that of men of the same age having no prostate cancer. The next logical step appears to be an investigation of the optimal duration of neoadjuvant combination therapy with flutamide and an LHRH superagonist before surgery. It is quite possible, as suggested by the use of an LHRH superagonist alone, that the inhibitory effect of androgen blockade could continue up to 6 months or longer [65] and that more beneficial effects could be obtained by increasing the duration of combination therapy before surgery. The potential advantages of continuing combination therapy after surgery to induce the death of cancer cells present in distant micrometastases in a significant proportion of patients at the start of therapy should also be investigated.

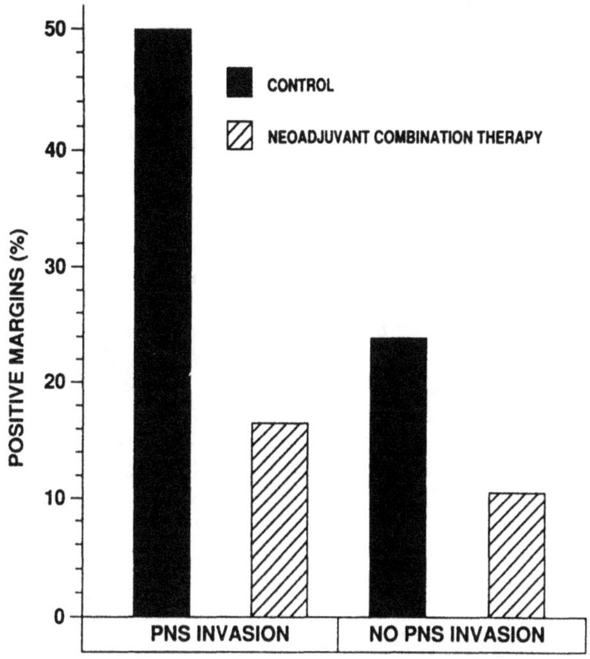

Fig. 8. Effect of 3-month neoadjuvant combination therapy with flutamide and an LHRH agonist on cancer-positive margins in 30 patients who had perineural space (PNS) invasion demonstrated after surgery compared with 36 patients not previously treated. In patients without PNS invasion, 24.1% (7/20) and 10.8% (5/46) had positive margins in the control and flutamide + LHRH agonist groups, respectively

REFERENCES

1 Huggins C and Hodges CV: Studies of prostatic cancer. I. Effect of castration, estrogen and androgen injections on serum phosphatases in metastatic carcinoma of the prostate. Cancer Res 1941 (1): 293-297

2 Veterans Administration Cooperative Urological Research Group (VACURG): Treatment and survival of patients with cancer of the prostate. Surg Gynecol Obstet 1967 (124):1011-1017

3 Labrie F, Dupont A and Bélanger A: A Complete androgen blockade for the treatment of prostate cancer. In: De Vita VT, Hellman S, Rosenberg SA (eds) Important Advances in Oncology. JB Lippincott, Philadelphia, 1985 pp 193-217

4 Labrie F: Intracrinology. Mol Cell Endocrinol 1991 (78):C-113-C118

5 Labrie F: Endocrine therapy of prostate cancer. Endocrinology and Metabolism Clinics of North America 1991 (20):845-872

6 Labrie F, Dupont A, Bélanger A et al: New hormonal therapy in prostatic carcinoma: combined treatment with an LHRH agonist and antiandrogen. J Clin Invest Med 1982 (5):267-275

7 Labrie F, Simard J, Luu-The V, Bélanger A, Pelletier G: Structure, function and tissue-specific gene expression of 3ß-hydroxysteroid dehydrogenase/5-ene-4-ene isomerase enzymes in classical and peripheral intracrine steroidogenic tissues. J Steroid Biochem Molec Biol 1992 (43):805-826

8 Labrie F, Bélanger A, Dupont A, Luu-The V, Simard J, Labrie C: Science behind total androgen blockade from gene to combination therapy. Clin Invest Med 1994 (in press)

9 Bélanger A, Brochu M, Cliche J: Levels of plasma steroid glucuronides in intact and castrated men with prostate cancer. J Clin Endocrinol Metab 1986 (62):812-815

10 Moghissi E, Ablan F, Horton R: Origin of plasma androstanediol glucuronide in men. J Clin Endocrinol Metab 1984 (59):417-421

11 Labrie F, Dupont A, Bélanger A et al: Treatment of prostate cancer with gonadotropin-releasing hormone agonists. Endocr Rev 1986 (7):67-74

12 Labrie F, Bélanger A, Cusan L et al: Antifertility effects of LHRH agonists in the male. J Androl 1980 (1):209-228

13 Neri R, Florance K, Koziol P, Van Cleave S: A biological profile of a non-steroidal antiandrogen, SCH 13521 (4'-nitro-3'-trifluoromethyl-isobutyranilide). Endocrinology 1972 (91):427-437

14 Poyet P and Labrie F: Comparison of the antiandrogenic/androgenic activities of flutamide, cyproterone acetate and megestrol acetate. Mol Cell Endocrinol 1985 (42):283-288

15 Labrie C, Cusan L, Plante M, Lapointe S, Labrie F: Analysis of the androgenic activity of synthetic "progestins" currently used for the treatment of prostate cancer. J Steroid Biochem 1987 (28):379-384

16 Labrie F and Veilleux R: A wide range of sensitivities to androgens develops in cloned Shionogi mouse mammary tumor cells. Prostate 1986 (8):293-300

17 Labrie F, Veilleux R, Fournier A: Low androgen levels induce the development of androgen hypersensitive cell clones in Shionogi mouse mammary carcinoma cells in culture. JNCI 1988 (80):1138-1147

18 Crawford ED, Eisenberger MA, McLeod DG et al: A controlled trial of leuprolide with and without flutamide in prostatic carcinoma. New Engl J Med 1989 (321):419-424

19 Denis L, Carneiro de Moura JL, Bono A, Sylvester R, Whelan P, Newling D, Depauw M and Members of the EORTC Group and EORTC Data center: Goserelin acetate and flutamide versus bilateral orchiectomy: a phase III EORTC Trial (30853). Urology 1993 (42):119-130

20 Soloway MS, Ishikawa S, van der Zwang R, Todd B: Prognostic factors in patients with advanced prostate cancer. Urology 1989 (33):53-56

21 Béland G, Elhilali M, Fradet Y et al: Total androgen blockade versus castration in metastatic cancer of the prostate. In: Motta M and Serio M (eds) Hormonal Therapy of Prostatic Diseases: Basic and Clinical Aspects. Medicom, Bussum 1988 pp 302-311

22 Janknegt RA, Abbou CC, Bartoletti R et al: Orchiectomy and Anandron (nilutamide) or placebo as treatment of metastatic prostatic cancer in a multinational double-blind randomized trial. Urology 1992 (149):77-83

23 Labrie F: GnRH agonists in prostate cancer. In: The Current Status of GnRH Analogues 1993, 3rd International Symposium on GnRH Analogues in Cancer and Human Reproduction, Parthenon Publishing, New York 1994 (in press)

24 Sanford EJ, Paulson DF, Rohner TJ, Drago JR, Santen RJ, Bardin CW: The effects of castration on adrenal testosterone secretion in men with prostatic carcinoma. J Urol 1977 (118):1019-1021

25 Rostom AY, Folkes A, Lord C, Notley RG, Schweitzer FAW, White WF: Aminoglutethimide therapy for advanced carcinoma of the prostate. Br J Urol 1982 (54):552-555

26 Labrie F, Dupont A, Giguère M et al: Important benefits of combination therapy with flutamide in patients relapsing after castration. Br J Urol 1988 (61):341-346

27 Labrie F, Dupont A, Bélanger A et al: Anti-hormone treatment for prostate cancer relapsing after treatment with flutamide and castration. Br J Urol 1989 (63):634-638

28 Eisenberger MA and Fontana JA: Suramin, an active nonhormonal cytotoxic drug for treatment of prostate cancer: compelling reasons for testing in patients with hormone-refractory breast cancer. JNCI 1992 (84):3-5

29 Belani CP, Pearl P, Whitley NO, Aisner J: Tamoxifen withdrawal response. Report of a case. Arch Intern Med 1989 (149):449-450

30 Rudolph RH: Response of metastatic breast cancer to tamoxifen (TAM) withdrawal, abstracted. In: Third European Conference on Clinical Oncology and Cancer Nursing, Stockholm 1981, p 161

31 Labrie F, Dupont A, Giguère M et al: Important prognostic value of standardized objective criteria of response in stage D2 prostatic carcinoma. Eur J Cancer Clin Oncol 1988 (12):1869-1878

32 Slack NH, Brady MF, Murphy GP and Investigators in the National Prostatic Cancer Project: Stable versus partial response in advanced prostate cancer. Prostate 1984 (5):401-415
33 Eisenberger MA, Simon R, O'Dwyer PJ, Winter RE, Friedman MA: A reevaluation of nonhormonal cytotoxic chemotherapy in the treatment of prostatic carcinoma. J Clin Oncol 1985 (3):827-841
34 Tannock IF: Is there evidence that chemotherapy is of benefit to patients with carcinoma of the prostate? J Clin Oncol 1985 (3):1013-1021
35 Schmidt JD, Mettlin CJ, Natarajan N, Peace B, Beart RW, Winchester DP, Murphy GP: Trends in patterns of care for prostatic cancer, 1974-1983; results of surveys by the American College of Surgeons. J Urol 1986 (136):416-421
36 Flocks RH, O'Donohue EPN, Milleman LA, Culp DA: Management of stage C prostatic carcinoma. Urol Clin North Amer 1975 (2):163-179
37 Paulson D, Hodge GB Jr, Hinshaw W: The Uro-Oncology Group. Radiation therapy versus delayed androgen de902privation for stage C carcinoma of the prostate. J Urol 1984 (131):901-902
38 Moorjani S, Dupont A, Labrie F et al: Increase in plasma high-density lipoprotein concentration following complete androgen blockage in men with prostatic carcinoma. Metabolism 1987 (36):244-250
39 Moorjani S, Dupont A, Labrie F et al: Changes in plasma lipoproteins during various androgen suppression therapies in men with prostatic carcinoma: effects of orchiectomy, estrogen and combination treatment with LHRH agonist and flutamide. J Clin Endocrinol Metab 1988 (66):314-322
40 Grayhack JT and Kozlowski JM: Endocrine therapy in the management of advanced prostatic cancer: the case for early initiation of treatment. Urol Clin North Amer 1980 (7):639-643
41 Kaplan EL and Meier P: Non parametric estimation from incomplete observations. J Am Stat Assoc 1958 (53):457-481
42 Whitmore WF Jr: The natural history of prostatic cancer. Cancer 1973 (32):1104-1112
43 Tomlinson RL, Currie DP, Boyce WH: Radical prostatectomy: palliation for stage C carcinoma of the prostate. J Urol 1977 (117):85-87
44 Dupont A, Gomez J-L, Cusan L, Koutsilieris M, Labrie F: Response to flutamide withdrawal in advanced prostate cancer in progression under combination therapy. J Urol 1993 (150):908-913
45 Cupps RE, Utz DC, Fleming TR, Carson CC, Zinckle H, Myers RP: Definitive radiation therapy for prostatic carcinoma: Mayo Clinic Experience. J Urol 1980 (124):855-859
46 Pavone-Macaluso M, de Voogt HJ, Viggiano G, Barasolo E, Lardennois B, de Pauw M, Sylvester R: Comparison of diethylstilbestrol, cyproterone acetate and medroxyprogesterone acetate in the treatment of advanced prostate cancer: final analysis of the randomized phase III trial of the European Organization for Research on Treatment of Cancer Urological Group. J Urol 1986 (136):624-631
47 Smith PH, Suciu S, Robinson MRG et al: A comparison of the effect of diethylstilbestrol with low dose estramustine phosphate in the treatment of advanced prostatic cancer: final analysis of a phase III of the European Organization for Research on Treatment of Cancer. J Urol 1986 (136):619-623
48 Catalona WJ and Bigg SW: Nerve-sparing radical prostatectomy: evaluation of results after 250 patients. J Urol 1990 (143):538-544
49 Epstein JI, Pizov G, Walsh PC: Correlation of pathologic findings with progression after radical retropubic prostatectomy. Cancer 1993 (71):3582-3593
50 Frazier HA, Robertson JE, Humphrey PA, Paulson DF: Is prostate specific antigen of clinical importance in evaluating outcome after radical prostatectomy? J Urol 1993 (149):516-518
51 Rosen MA, Goldstone L, Lapin S, Wheeler T, Scardino PT: Frequency and location of extracapsular extension and positive surgical margins in radical prostatectomy specimens. J Urol 1992 (148):331-337
52 Stein A, De Kernion JB, Smith RB, Dorey F, Patel H: Prostate specific antigen levels after radical prostatectomy in patients with organ-confined and locally extensive prostate cancer. J Urol 1992 (147):942-946
53 Brendler CB, Carmichael M, Walsh PC, Epstein JI: Radical prostatectomy for nonpalpable prostate cancer diagnosed by needle biopsy: pathologic and clinical findings. J Urol 1993 (149):378A
54 Andros EA, Danesghari F, Crawford ED: Neoadjuvant hormonal therapy in stage C carcinoma of the prostate. Clin Invest Med 1994 (in press)
55 Fair WR, Aprikian A, Cohen D, Sogani P, Reuter V: The use of neoadjuvant androgen deprivation therapy in clinically localized prostate cancer. Clin Invest Med 1993 (in press)
56 Lee F, Siders DB, Newby JE, McHugh TA, Solomon MH: The role of transrectal ultrasound guided staging biopsy and androgen ablation therapy prior to radical prostatectomy. Clin Invest Med 1994 (in press)
57 McHugh TA: The influence of transrectal ultrasound of the prostate on a private urology practice. In: Labrie F, Lee F, Dupont A (eds) Early Stage Prostate Cancer: Diagnosis and Choice of Therapy. Excerpta Medica, New York 1989 pp 37-40
58 Monfette G, Dupont A, Labrie F: Temporary combination therapy with flutamide and Tryptex as adjuvant to radical prostatectomy for the treatment of early stage prostate cancer. In: Labrie F, Lee F, Dupont A (eds) Early Stage Prostate Cancer: Diagnosis and Choice of Therapy. Excerpta Medica, New York 1989 pp 41-42
59 Solomon MH, McHugh T, Door RP, Lee F, Siders DB: Hormone ablation therapy as neoadjuvant treatment to radical prostatectomy. Clin Invest Med 1994 (in press)
60 Têtu B, Srigley Jr, Boivin JC: Effect of combination endocrine therapy (LHRH agonist and flutamide) on normal prostate and prostatic adenocarcinoma: a histopathologic and immunohisto-chemical study. Am J Surg Pathol 1991 (15):111-120
61 Labrie F, Dupont A, Cusan L et al: Downstaging of localized prostate cancer by neoadjuvant therapy with flutamide and lupron. Clin Invest Med 1994 (in press)
62 Byar DP and Mostofi FK: Carcinoma of the prostate: prognostic evaluation of certain pathologic features

in 208 radical prostatectomies. Examined by step-section technique. Cancer 1972 (30):5-13
63 Villers A, McNeal JE, Redwine EA, Freiha FS, Stamey TA: The radical perineural space invasion in the local spread of prostatic adenocarcinoma. J Urol 1989 (142):763-768
64 Brendler CB and Walsh PC: The role of radical prostatectomy in the treatment of prostate cancer. CA Cancer J Clin 1992 (42):212-222
65 Botto H, Richard F, Mathieu F, Camey M: Decapeptyl in the treatment of advanced prostatic cancer: comparative study with pulpectomy. Prog Clin Biol Res 1989 (303):53-60
66 Labrie F, Dupont A, Simard J, Luu-The V, Bélanger A: Intracrinology: The basis for the rational design of endocrine therapy at all stages of prostate cancer. Eur Urol 1993 ( ):94-105

Casodex*: Preclinical Studies

Barry J.A. Furr

Vascular, Inflammatory and Musculoskeletal Research Department, ZENECA Pharmaceuticals, Alderley Park, Macclesfield, Cheshire SK10 4TG, United Kingdom

The established treatment for prostate cancer is endocrine manipulation since the growth of a majority of prostate tumours is stimulated by the male sex hormones, androgens. Thus, effective withdrawal of androgen by orchidectomy or oestrogen therapy has been the major form of treatment for prostate cancer for several decades. Orchidectomy is unpopular with patients, causes a loss of libido and can result in psychological trauma; since it is ineffective in about one quarter of patients they will have been submitted to unnecessary surgery. Although oestrogen therapy is effective in a majority of patients it is associated with unacceptably high morbidity and mortality, apparently due to cardiovascular complications, so survival is not increased [1]. As well as increasing the incidence of thromboembolism and causing fluid retention, oestrogen treatment also leads to the development of painful and embarrassing gynaecomastia and a loss of libido [2,3].

In the last decade, luteinising hormone-releasing hormone (LHRH) agonist analogues have been used to produce a "medical" castration for the treatment of prostate cancer [4-6]. Long acting depot formulations of these drugs have now been developed, for example, Zoladex [5, 7], which overcome the problems of daily parenteral dosing and its associated compliance difficulties. More recently, combination of LHRH agonist with an antiandrogen, a treatment termed "total androgen withdrawal", has been shown in some studies to be superior to LHRH agonists alone [8,9]. However, all of these procedures either only lead to the withdrawal of androgen produced by the testes or require combination therapy.

A drug which antagonises the action of any androgen, whether produced by the gonad or adrenal glands, would also be useful for the treatment of prostate cancer. Three such antiandrogenic drugs (Fig. 1) have been used clinically. Cyproterone acetate, the first antiandrogen to be used clinically, is a tribute to the pioneering work of Neumann and colleagues at Schering AG. Cyproterone acetate is a steroidal antiandrogen which is effective in a majority of patients and produces side-effects which are generally less than those seen with oestrogens [3]. However, thrombosis is seen in 5% of patients, fluid retention in 4%, gynaecomastia in 13% and loss of libido in the majority; the steroidal nature of the drug is probably responsible for its cardiovascular side-effects and its adverse effect on serum lipoproteins [10]. Because of its steroidal properties there can be effects on carbohydrate metabolism so care is advised when prescribing the drug for diabetic patients [11,12]. Variable degrees of migraine and gastrointestinal upset have been reported [3]. Cyproterone acetate is also a potent progestin. The progestational properties of cyproterone acetate provide an advantage over surgical and medical castration and some antiandrogens because the drug does not produce hot flushes. However, cyproterone acetate does severely suppress libido and causes gynaecomastia and loss of erectile potency [13]. Loss of libido may not be a severe disadvantage in many very old patients but in younger men with prostate cancer who are sexually active, loss of libido would be an unfavourable consequence of therapy.

Flutamide, the first available non-steroidal antiandrogen, was a very significant discovery

* Casodex and Zoladex are trade marks of ZENECA Limited

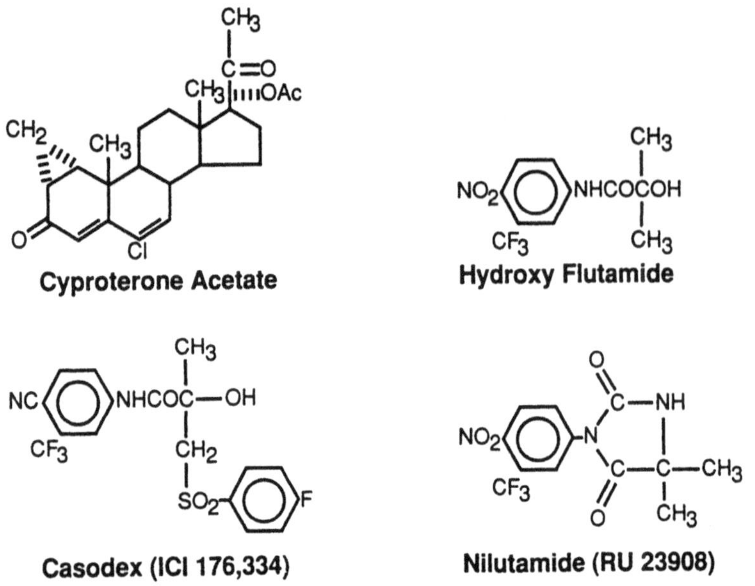

Fig. 1. Structures of antiandrogens

by Neri and colleagues at Schering-Plough. Flutamide is also effective in the treatment of prostate cancer and appears to be better tolerated than cyproterone acetate [3]. Since it is a pure antiandrogen, it does not seem to be associated with the side-effects of thromboembolism and fluid retention. Moreover, since it is not a progestin it does not suppress testis function like cyproterone acetate and it rarely causes a loss of libido. Gynaecomastia is the most frequently reported side-effect [3], but gastrointestinal intolerance, particularly diarrhoea, can be a troublesome side-effect in some patients [14,15]. Reversible liver function abnormalities have been reported in some patients which can sometimes be serious [16]. The active metabolite of flutamide, hydroxyflutamide, also has a short half-life (5.2 hours) and so the parent drug needs to be administered 3 times daily [17], which may lead to problems with compliance with therapy. Since it is a pure antiandrogen there is another perceived problem with flutamide: as well as preventing androgen from stimulating prostate growth, it antagonises the action of androgen at the hypothalamus and pituitary gland. This leads to an increase in luteinising hormone (LH) secretion. It is suggested that the resulting increase in output of androgen by the testis requires an increased dose of antiandrogen to neutralise any stimulatory effect on the prostate gland. This is a controversial topic which will be discussed further later in this chapter. In addition to elevating androgen secretion, serum oestrogen concentrations are also increased, which would tend to exacerbate any tendency to gynaecomastia.

Nilutamide, the second non-steroidal pure antiandrogen to become available from Roussel, is structually similar to flutamide, but has a longer half-life (approximately 2 days) [18], so it can theoretically be given once daily. Clinical trials with nilutamide have focussed primarily on its combination with surgical or medical castration [9,19]. The side-effects of the drug include problems with light-dark adaptation [19-21], interstitial pneumonitis [19], which reportedly led to clinical trial cessation in Japan, and alcohol intolerance [19].

It is the objective of research-based pharmaceutical companies to discover new therapies for disease that have readily discernible advantages over existing drugs. Thus, at Zeneca we concluded that a potent, pure antiandrogen that was well tolerated and had a half-life compatible with once daily dosing would offer clinical advantages over the existing therapies, since libido should be maintained, compliance with therapy would be less of an issue and tolerance should be good. In addition, it was hoped that a peripherally selective antiandrogen could be identified that would prevent prostate growth but would not act at the hypothalamic-pituitary gonadal axis to increase serum LH and thereby testosterone. Casodex (ICI 176,334, see Fig. 1) [22] was identified from over 1000 compounds synthesized for this purpose as having such desirable properties. The pharmacodynamic properties of Casodex that support this expectation are the subject of this chapter.

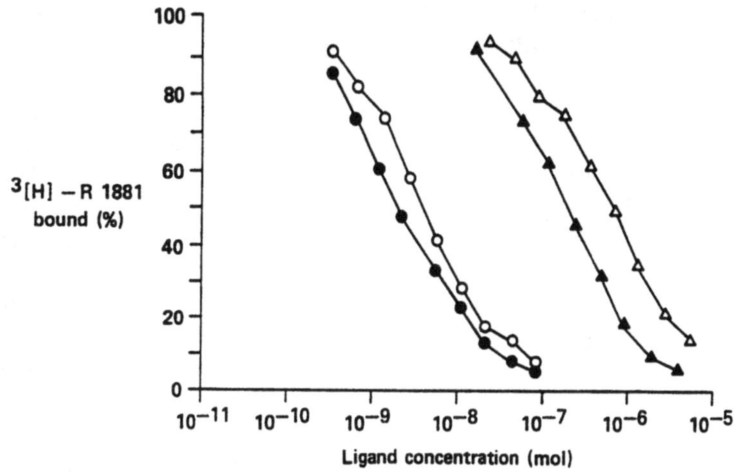

Fig. 2. Displacement of [3H]-R1881 from a rat prostate androgen receptor preparation by increasing concentration of unlabelled R1881 (●---●), 5α-dihydrotestosterone (○---○), Casodex (▲---▲) and hydroxyflutamide (Δ---Δ)

Receptor Binding Studies

Preliminary studies investigated binding of Casodex to rat prostate cytosol androgen receptors. Displacement curves using cold drugs and the potent selective androgen [^{3}H]-R1881 are shown in Figure 2.

Both 5α-dihydrotestosterone and R1881 have much higher affinity for the receptor than the antiandrogens, with Casodex being superior to hydroxyflutamide. This is reinforced by the IC_{50} values (mass of compound which causes 50% displacement of specifically bound radioligand) for the 4 compounds and the percentage crossreactivity of the 3 synthetic compounds compared with the natural ligand, 5α-dihydrotestosterone (Table 1).

These results have been confirmed by Winneker, Wagner and Batzold [23], who showed that Casodex had a relative binding affinity of 2% compared with R1881 (100%) after 1 hour incubation and 0.43% after 18 hours incubation. Similarly, Casodex was shown to bind to a stable transfectant of the rat androgen receptor and MMTV-CAT (mouse mammary tumour virus chloramphenicol acetyltransferase) and to block the effects of R1881; Casodex alone was devoid of agonist activity [24]. Casodex also binds to rat pituitary cytosol androgen receptors with similar relative affinity as well as to dog and human prostate androgen receptors.

Juniewicz et al. [25] described the binding of Casodex to the adult beagle dog prostate androgen receptor. Similar relative binding affinities to R1881 were found to those described above for the rat receptor. Cyproterone acetate had a higher affinity than Casodex but that of hydroxyflutamide was lower. All of the antiandrogens had significantly lower binding affinities than 5α-dihydrotestosterone.

Two studies in the literature describe the binding of Casodex to human prostate androgen receptor [26,27]. Ayub and Levell [26] compared the relative affinities of cyproterone acetate, Casodex, nilutamide and hydroxyflutamide for the human androgen receptor obtained from hyperplastic prostates. Casodex was found to bind to the human prostate androgen receptor with an affinity lower than the potent androgens, R1881 and 5α-dihydrotestosterone, but with a higher relative affinity than nilutamide and hydroxyflutamide.

In this study, Casodex was also shown to have negligible affinity for sex hormone-binding globulin and no affinity for corticosteroid-binding globulin. In contrast, cyproterone acetate had significant affinity for sex hormone-binding globulin and high affinity (36% relative to control = 100%) for corticosteroid-binding globulin.

Casodex also bound to human androgen receptors transfected into COS cells both in the native form and with a point mutation (codon 868, threonine to alanine) derived from LNCaP

Table 1. Prostate androgen receptor binding data

Compound	IC50 (nMol)	% Cross-reaction
R1881	2	190
5α-dihydrotestosterone	3.8	100
Casodex	190	2
Hydroxyflutamide	700	0.5

human prostate tumour cells [27]. Again, Casodex had a low affinity (0.3%) compared with R1881 (100%) and 5α-dihydrotestosterone (33%) but had comparable affinity to hydroxyflutamide (0.4%) and nilutamide (0.1%) for the normal receptor.

It should be emphasized that Casodex has no effect on steroid 5α-reductase [28].

Effects of Casodex on Tumour Cells in Vitro

An important study by Veldscholte et al. [29] describes the effects of Casodex on binding to an androgen receptor present in the human LNCaP prostate tumour cell line. In this tumour line, the androgen receptor has a point mutation in the steroid-binding domain (Codon 868, Thr to Ala). This defect does not prevent antiandrogens like cyproterone acetate, nilutamide and hydroxyflutamide from binding to the receptor but the resulting receptor complex *stimulates* growth of the cell line: it does not prevent androgen-induced growth. Casodex is unique amongst currently available antiandrogens in that it does *not* stimulate cell growth. Casodex will, however, inhibit growth in response to the synthetic androgen R1881. Hydroxyflutamide only stimulates cell growth in these experiments.

Detailed molecular biology work showed that the heat shock proteins Hsp90, 70 and 56 coprecipitate with the androgen receptor and so may have a chaperon role. Binding of androgens and the older antiandrogens with the receptor caused dissociation of the heat shock proteins and, in parallel, transformation of the receptor to a tight nuclear-binding form. In contrast, Casodex did not cause dissociation of the associated heat shock proteins and transformation of the androgen receptor to a tight nuclear-binding form did not occur. Whether this observation has any clinical significance must await the outcome of further studies but it is tempting to speculate that Casodex would still be effective in some tumours which fail to respond to primary therapy with other antiandrogens or that it may be effective in tumours relapsing on such antiandrogen therapy. Evidence that some patients show withdrawal responses to flutamide is now available [30,31]: such tumours might actually be stimulated by flutamide if they arise from cell clones that contain a mutated androgen receptor but would still be responsive to Casodex. Examination of androgen receptors by PCR and sequence analysis from refractory and relapsing patients would help to determine whether this conjecture is valid.

The Shionogi S115 mouse mammary tumour cell line contains androgen receptors and its growth can be stimulated by androgens [32]. Short-term androgen withdrawal results in a change from fibroblastic to epithelial morphology, reduced proliferation rate, increased density regulation and the loss of ability to grow in suspension culture [33]. Long-term growth of these cells in the absence of androgen also results in an ordered, reproducible series of phenotypic changes culminating in loss of both cellular and gene-sensitive markers responsive to androgen. Darbre and King [33] have described the effects of Casodex on this cell line. Casodex (10^{-6}M) inhibited cell growth stimulation by testosterone (10^{-9}M) in monolayer cultures and was particularly effective against testosterone at 10^{-8}M. Similarly, Casodex at 10^{-6}M prevented the growth of suspension cultures of SC-115 cells in the presence of testosterone (10^{-9}M) and the proliferation of mouse mammary tumour virus RNA.

Casodex had no agonist activity at 10^{-6}M since it failed to promote growth in either monolayer of suspension culture and the cells were of an epithelial appearance. Moreover, Casodex had no stimulatory effect on mouse mammary tumour virus RNA production whereas androgen did cause such a stimulation.

There are also 3 literature reports of the effects of Casodex on cells transfected with androgen receptors. Fuhrmann et al. [24] stably transfected the rat androgen receptor and a mouse mammary tumour virus, chloramphenicol acetyltransferase (MMTV-CAT) gene construct into receptor-negative CV-1 cells. In contrast to the potent androgen R1881, neither hydroxyflutamide nor Casodex stimulated CAT activity. Both non-steroidal antiandrogens inhibited, in a dose-dependent manner, CAT expression induced by R1881.

Veldscholte et al. [27,29] have described the effects of Casodex on a HeLa cell line stably transfected with either the normal human androgen receptor (wild type) or the receptor with a point mutation (Codon 868, Thr to Ala) found in the LNCaP prostate tumour cell line. A glucocorticoid-responsive element linked to chlorma-

Table 2. Effects of daily administration of Casodex (10 mg/kg s.c.) and flutamide (2 mg/kg p.o.) on accessory sex organ weights in groups of 5 immature castrated rats given testosterone propionate (200 µg/kg/day) concurrently. Values are expressed as mg/100 g body weight and % inhibition (maximum inhibition (100%) is taken as the value for historical data in castrated animals not given testosterone propionate)

Treatment	Seminal Vesicles		Ventral Prostate	
	mg/100 g	% Inhibition	mg/100 g	% Inhibition
Testosterone propionate (TP)	21.61 ± 1.35	0	36.45 ± 2.78	0
Placebo control	6	100	14.7	100
Flutamide + TP	10.70 ± 0.44***	73.9	29.69 ± 2.45***	31.1
Casodex + TP	5.78 ± 0.22+++***	101.4	15.43 ±1.22+++***	96.6

*** $p < 0.001$ compared with TP alone
+++ $p < 0.001$ compared with TP + flutamide

phenicol acetyl transferase (CAT), pG29Gtk CAT was used as a reporter. Casodex failed to stimulate CAT activity in either transfected cell line and inhibited CAT expression induced by R1881. Hydroxyflutamide behaved as a pure antiandrogen in the cell line containing the wild type construct but stimulated CAT expression in the cell line containing the mutated receptor without being able to inhibit CAT activity induced by R1881. Thus, these results are in accord with the findings in the LNCaP cell line [29].

Antiandrogenic Effects of Casodex in Male Rats

The effects of Casodex in immature castrated rats treated daily with testosterone propionate (200 µg/kg) are shown in Table 2. Casodex produces a profound inhibition of androgen-stimulated accessory sex organ growth and at a dose of 10 mg/kg is significantly more active than flutamide. Dose response studies show that Casodex produces a significant inhibition of testosterone propionate-induced accessory sex organ growth at oral doses down to 0.25 mg/kg. These findings were supported by studies in castrated immature male rats given a higher dose of testosterone propionate (0.8 or 1 mg/kg) [34], where Casodex was more potent than flutamide, cyproterone acetate and WIN 49,596, a new steroidal antiandrogen.

A comparison of the oral activity of Casodex and flutamide was made in mature male rats (200-220 g) with a 14-day dosing period followed by necropsy on day 15. The doses used and results obtained are shown in Figure 3. Casodex reduced the weights of the seminal vesicles and ventral prostate glands at all of the dose levels tested but did not cause a significant elevation in either LH or testosterone at any dose. In contrast, flutamide caused dose-related increases in both serum LH and testosterone.

These results have been confirmed and extended by a report from Snyder, Winneker and Batzold [34], and 3 studies by Nieschlag's group. Snyder, Winneker and Batzold [34] compared the effects of Casodex (15 mg/kg), flutamide (15 mg/kg) and WIN 49,596 (100 mg/kg) on serum testosterone after 7 and 14 days of treatment. Both Casodex and WIN 49,596 caused a small (2-3 fold) increase in serum testosterone concentrations whereas flutamide caused a larger (7-11 fold) increase in serum testosterone. These results are essentially equivalent to the studies on Casodex reported here, where flutamide always causes a marked and highly significant increase in LH, whereas Casodex causes a small, usually non-significant, increase in the serum concentrations of this gonadotrophin.

Chandolia et al. [35] showed that daily oral doses of Casodex of 10, 20 and 40 mg/kg for 14 days failed to increase serum testosterone concentrations although the highest dose caused a significant increase in testis testosterone content; flutamide (10 mg/kg) did cause a significant elevation in serum testosterone. The two lower doses of Casodex affected neither serum LH nor FSH concentrations but the highest dose did cause a small but significant increase in serum LH only, at day 15. In

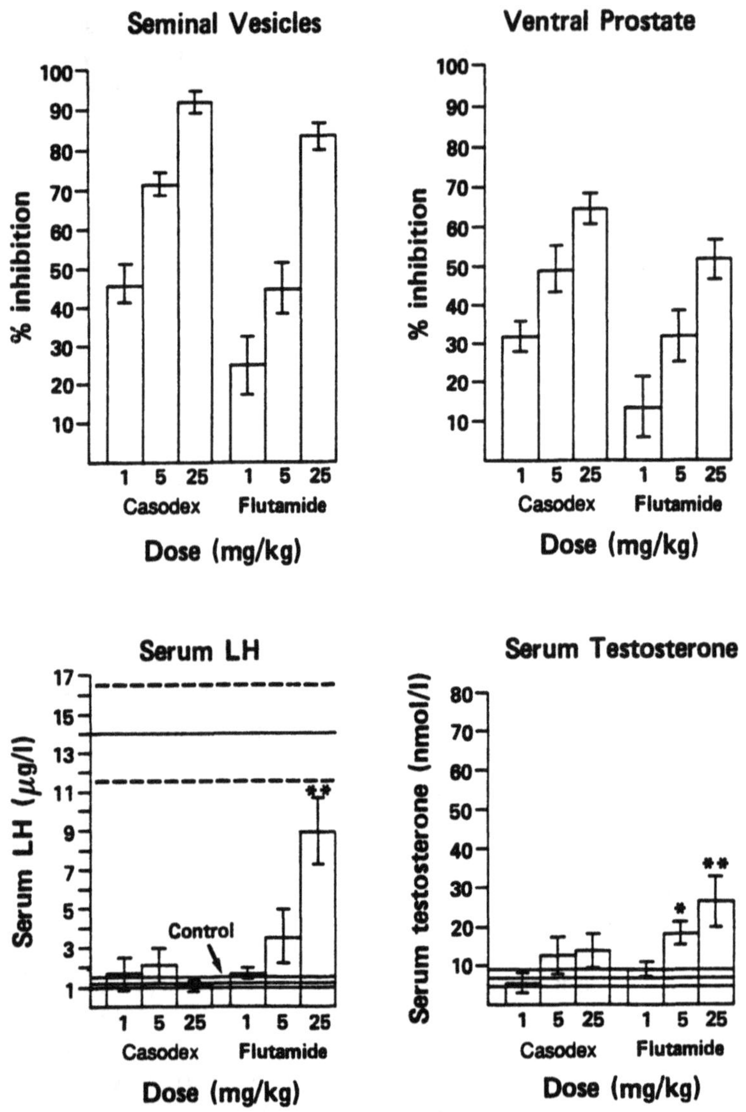

Fig. 3. Comparison of the effects of graded oral doses of flutamide and Casodex administered daily for 14 days on weights of the seminal vesicles and ventral prostate glands and on serum LH and serum testosterone levels in mature male rats. Placebo-treated controls are arbitrarily assigned a value of 0 and surgically castrated controls a value of 100% for measuring inhibition of organ weights. Solid horizontal lines show the range of hormone values for placebo-treated controls and dashed lines the value for surgically castrated controls.
*$p < 0.05$; **$p < 0.01$ compared with placebo-treated control values

contrast, flutamide caused highly significant elevations in LH at all time points and a progressive significant elevation in FSH. Interestingly, pituitary gonadotrophin concentrations were unaltered by Casodex treatment whilst flutamide induced a decrease in pituitary LH. In these studies, Casodex also caused significant decreases in seminal vesicle and epididymal weights at all dose levels but no change in testes or pituitary gland weights. However, in contrast to flutamide, Casodex caused a significant loss of germ cells in stage VII of spermatogenesis and enhanced spermatogenic involution caused by an LHRH antagonist. These findings are consistent with the view that Casodex is a more potent antiandrogen than flutamide.

Chandolia et al. [36] confirmed and extended these studies by administering Casodex orally to rats for 3 and 8 weeks at 20 mg/kg and comparing with flutamide (20 mg/kg). The results showed again that Casodex was a more potent antiandrogen than flutamide and caused no increase in serum testosterone and only a small elevation in serum LH compared with the marked and highly significant elevations in these hormones produced following treatment with flutamide.

In a third paper, Simoni et al. [37] showed that oral Casodex at 20 mg/kg for 8 weeks caused no changes in serum immunoreactive or bioactive FSH, a small increase in pituitary immunoreactive FSH but no changes in serum inhibin and testosterone concentrations. In contrast, flutamide significantly elevated serum immunoreactive and bioactive FSH had no effect on pituitary FSH but significantly elevated both serum testosterone and inhibin. This is an

unusual finding because serum inhibin and FSH normally show a reciprocal relationship.
It can be concluded that all of the independent published work confirms the view that Casodex is a potent antiandrogen that is peripherally selective. In contrast, flutamide has lower potency and no peripheral selectivity in rats.

Studies to Define the Reasons for the Peripheral Selectivity of Casodex in Male Rats

A number of possible reasons for the peripheral selectivity of Casodex were apparent. Firstly, there was the possibility that the androgen receptors present in the pituitary gland and hypothalamus were different. This remains a possibility but molecular biological studies in several laboratories have failed, so far, to demonstrate multiple androgen receptors. Moreover, the data described above demonstrate that Casodex binds as effectively to the pituitary androgen receptor as it does to the ventral prostate receptor. A second explanation could be that when bound to the pituitary androgen receptor some subtle mechanism comes into play which masks the expected antiandrogenic response. Since both Casodex and flutamide are equally effective at sensitizing the pituitary gland to the LHRH agonist Zoladex (Fig. 4), this explanation cannot be valid.
A third explanation is that the hypothalamic androgen receptor behaves differently from the peripheral androgen receptors, including that in the pituitary gland. This is unlikely to be the case since Belchetz [38] showed that Casodex increased LHRH pulse frequency in rat hypothalamic fragments *in vitro* and that both Casodex and hydroxyflutamide increased LHRH pulse frequency following suppression with testosterone. Hence, both of these compounds behave as intrinsic antiandrogens at the hypothalamic androgen receptor.
A further explanation is that Casodex penetrates the blood-brain barrier poorly and thus fails to achieve adequate concentrations in the hypothalamus needed to exert marked antiandrogenic effects. This is indeed the case as tissue distribution studies with [3H]-Casodex have shown [39] (Fig. 5).
The tissues studied can be divided into 5 major groups on the basis of how they sequester

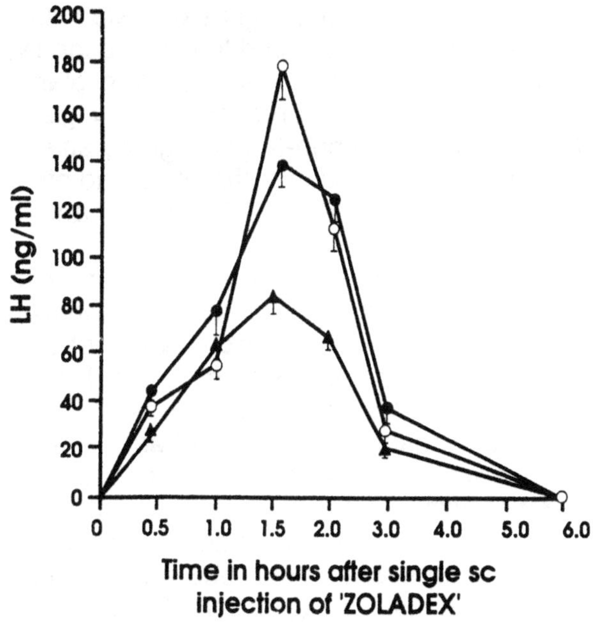

Fig. 4. Effect of 0.1 μg Zoladex s.c. on serum LH in male rats pretreated for 14 days with either 0.5% polysorbate p.o. (▲---▲), 5 mg flutamide/kg p.o. (●---●) or 5 mg Casodex/kg p.o. (○---○). The values shown are the means ± sem, N=5

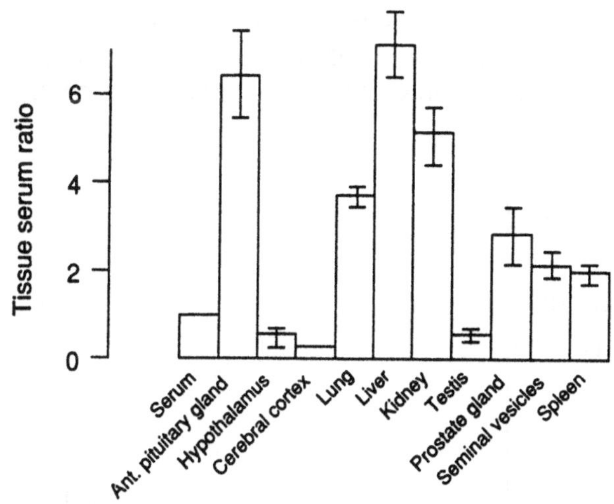

Fig. 5. Distribution of radioactivity in the intact male rat following intravenous injection of ^{3}H Casodex. Rats were killed 1 hour after injection and tissues were solubilised and counted for tritium. Tissue radioactivity was expressed as dpm mg -1 tissue weight and then as a tissue-to-serum ratio (TSR). Histogram height reflects the mean TSR for each tissue in each group (n = 4 or 5); the vertical lines represent the standard errors of the means

radioactivity. Firstly the organs of metabolism and excretion, the liver and kidney; secondly, the androgen target tissues, prostate gland, seminal vesicles and anterior pituitary gland (APG); thirdly, the non-target organs, spleen and lung; fourthly, the hypothalamus and other central nervous system (CNS) tissues; and finally the testes.

The mean hepatic and renal tissue to serum ratios (TSRs) 1, 5 or 10 hours following injection of [^{3}H]-Casodex were significantly higher ($p < 0.05$) than the corresponding means for the prostate gland and spleen. The mean TSRs for the target organs prostate gland and seminal vesicles were not significantly different from the corresponding splenic mean at any of the 3 times after injection. As expected from the *in vitro* binding studies described earlier, there was substantial uptake of [^{3}H]-Casodex by the anterior pituitary gland (APG).

Mean testis TSR was seen to be significantly lower ($p < 0.05$) than the corresponding splenic means 1 hour after injection. No such significant differences were demonstrable either 5 hours or 10 hours after injection of [^{3}H]-Casodex.

The mean hypothalamic and cerebrocortical TSRs 1 hour, 5 hours and 10 hours after injection were an order of magnitude lower than the corresponding means for any of the other tissues studied, indicating that Casodex penetrates poorly into the central nervous system.

Antitumour Effects of Casodex in Rats

Studies on the antitumour effects of Casodex were carried out in rats bearing the Dunning R3327H prostate tumour.

In the first experiment groups of 10 animals were given daily oral doses of either 0.5% polysorbate or Casodex (25 mg/kg). Two further groups of 10 animals were surgically castrated and given identical control and drug treatments. The tumour growth response is shown in Figure 6. Tumours in the intact control group grew rapidly. Castration and Casodex treatment caused significant ($p < 0.05$) suppression of growth with all of these treatments producing responses of a similar magnitude; there was no significant difference in tumour growth rate in castrated rats and castrated rats given Casodex.

In another experiment, the efficacy of Casodex was compared with flutamide. The drugs were given as daily oral doses at both 25 and 5 mg/kg in groups of 8 animals. In this experiment, dosing was continued until the tumour size in individual animals reached 20 cm^2 when they were killed; serum was collected for radioimmunoassay of FSH, LH and testosterone. The treated groups could be compared with the intact control groups for the first 11 weeks of study only. The results are shown in Figure 7. Casodex caused a significant ($p < 0.05$, weeks

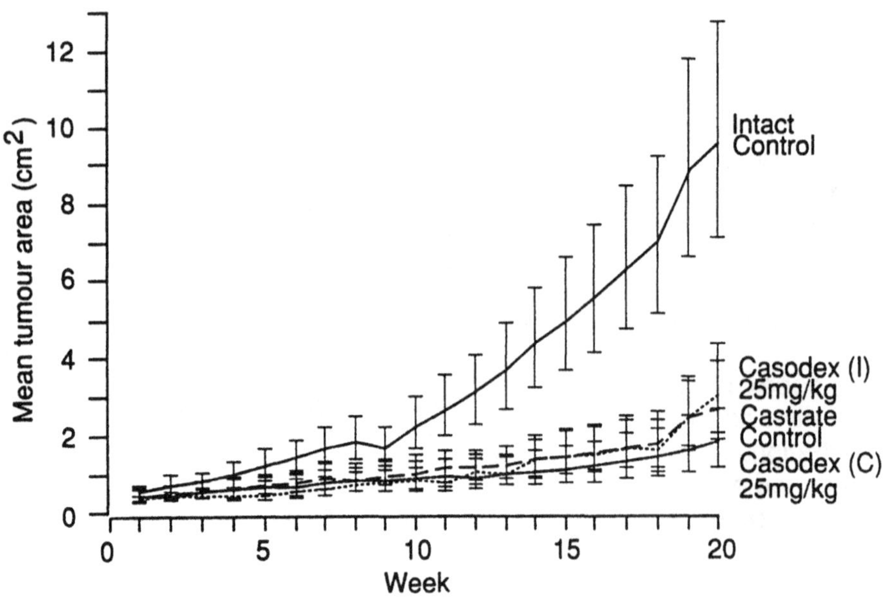

Fig. 6. Effect of a daily oral dose of 25 mg Casodex/kg on the growth of Dunning prostate tumours. I = intact; C = castrate

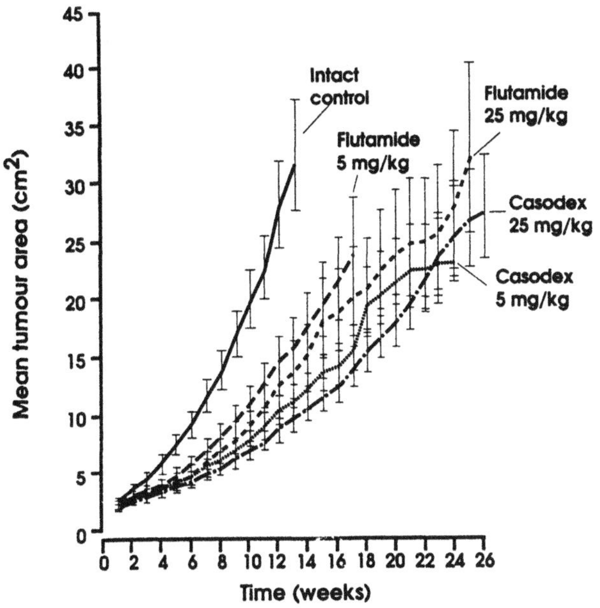

Fig. 7. Comparison of the effects of Casodex and flutamide at daily oral doses of 5 and 25 mg/kg on growth of Dunning prostate tumours

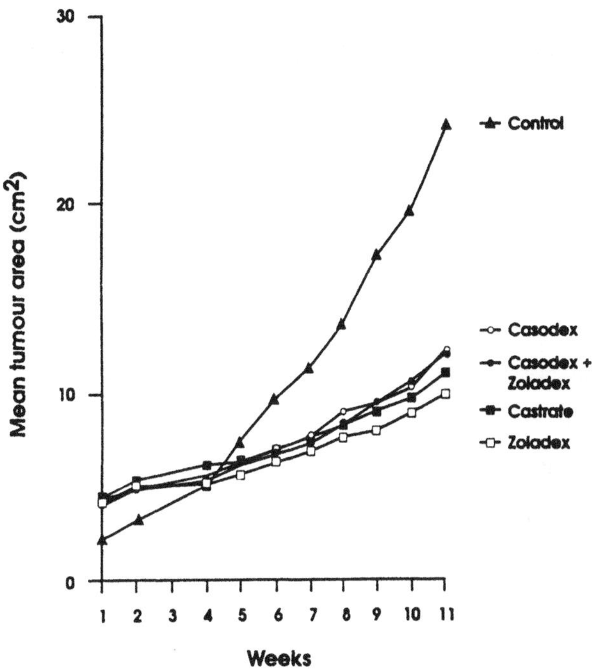

Fig. 8. Effect of single s.c. 1 mg Zoladex depots given every 28 days, daily oral administration of 25 mg Casodex/kg and the combination of both treatments on the growth of Dunning prostate tumours. The effects of surgical castration at the start of the experiment are also shown

4-5; $p < 0.01$ weeks 6-11) inhibition in tumour growth rate at both 5 and 25 mg/kg with no difference in the response achieved by either of these doses. Flutamide appeared less effective but produced a significant ($p < 0.05$) reduction in tumour size at weeks 6-11 at a dose of 25 mg/kg and at weeks 7-11 at a dose of 5 mg/kg. Even at the higher dose the mean effect was not as great as that seen with Casodex at 5 mg/kg.

In this study, an analysis was performed of the time taken for the total tumour size to increase to an ethically acceptable maximum level (≥20 cm^2) or to death if this occurred earlier. Survival time was significantly shorter for intact controls than for drug-treated animals (flutamide (25 mg/kg), p=0.015; flutamide (5 mg/kg), p=0.029; Casodex (25 mg/kg), p=0.007; Casodex (5 mg/ kg), p=0.016).

Since the animals were killed at different times during the experiment, caution must be exercised in the interpretation of organ weight data. However, it is clear that Casodex is considerably more potent than flutamide at causing regression of the accessory sex organs. Moreover, Casodex fails to affect serum LH and testosterone, in contrast to flutamide which elevates both hormones even at the lower dose of 5 mg/kg

In view of the interest in the concept of "total androgen withdrawal" [40], a comparison was made of the effects of treatment with single subcutaneous biodegradable depots containing 1 mg of the LHRH agonist Zoladex [41] given every 28 days, daily oral administration of Casodex (25 mg/kg), and combination of the two therapies in rats bearing Dunning prostate tumours. The results are shown in Figure 8 and clearly indicate that both Zoladex and Casodex treatment alone are as effective as surgical castration at inhibiting the growth rate of these prostate tumours. Furthermore, there is no advantage of the combination therapy over the single therapies.

Zoladex produces the expected castration effect on serum testosterone and accessory sex organ weights, which is not altered by the addition of Casodex. Since adrenal androgen contributes little to circulating androgens in the male rat, these findings should not be used to cast doubt on the validity of the total androgen withdrawal hypothesis.

The endocrine data are entirely consistent with the previous findings. Casodex causes a highly significant reduction in accessory sex organ

Table 3. Effect of Casodex on histological appearance of testes, epididymides and prostate in adult male beagle dogs

	Dose of CASODEX (mg/kg)					
	0	0.25	0.5	1	2	4
Atrophy of Prostate						
None	5	0	0	0	0	0
Mild	0	1	0	0	0	0
Moderate	0	1	1	0	0	0
Marked	0	3	4	5	3	5
Atrophy of Testes						
None	5	5	5	3	5	2
Mild	0	0	0	0	0	0
Moderate	0	0	0	2	0	3
Atrophy of Epididymides						
None	5	4	2	0	0	0
Mild	0	1	3	5	4	2
Moderate	0	0	0	0	1	3

weights but these did not quite achieve castrate values. Serum FSH is slightly stimulated by treatment with Casodex but there is no significant effect on serum LH, prolactin and testosterone.

Endocrine Effects of Casodex in Dogs

The effects of oral administration of Casodex daily for 6 weeks were evaluated in adult male beagle dogs; doses ranged from 0.25 to 4 mg/kg. No change in the clinical condition or the behaviour of the animals was noted and the only clinically relevant finding at necropsy was a reduction in size of the testes, epididymides and prostate gland. This observation was confirmed by the assessment of organ weights: testes, epididymides and prostate weights were all decreased by treatment. There is, however, a large variation in prostate size in control dogs of this age range, so the histological effects give a clearer guide to the efficacy of Casodex.

Table 3 shows that Casodex caused atrophy of the prostate gland and epididymides at all dose levels and testis atrophy in 3 out of 5 dogs at the highest dose level (4 mg/kg) and in 2 out of 5 at 1 mg/kg.

Since 0.25 mg/kg was above the ED_{50} dose for Casodex, the study was repeated using an identical protocol except that doses of 0.25, 0.1 and 0.05 mg Casodex/kg were used. No clinically relevant findings were noted. At necropsy the weight of the prostate glands in all drug dosed groups was lower than that of the controls; there were no clear effects on weights of testis or epididymides. Histological examination showed that atrophy of the prostate was dose related with 0.1 mg/kg being an approximate ED_{50}. Atrophy of the epididymides was less marked and was only seen in tissue from dogs given 0.25 mg Casodex/kg. There were no significant effects on serum testosterone concentrations. Indeed, estimation of serum testosterone concentrations from a sighting toxicity study where daily oral doses of 20 and 100 mg Casodex/kg were given for 28 days shows that even at these doses, which are very substantial multiples of the ED_{50} value, there is no effect on serum testosterone concentrations. These results are in accord with the findings in beagle dogs of Juniewicz et al. [25], who showed that an oral dose of Casodex (0.25 mg/kg) daily caused a significant reduction in prostate volume assessed by ultrasound at 2 weeks after the start of treatment and was more potent than the steroidal antiandrogen WIN 49596 and the 5α-reductase inhibitor MK-906. After 16 weeks of treatment, Casodex (0.25 mg/kg daily orally) also induced a significant reduction in prostate weights and prostate DNA content compared with intact controls but this dose was not equivalent to surgical castra-

in dogs treated with Casodex and there was a significant reduction in semen volume after 16 weeks of treatment with Casodex [25].

There was also no effect of Casodex on testes weights at 0.25 mg/kg daily nor on spermatogenesis and Leydig cell appearance. Finally, Juniewicz et al. [25] confirmed the ZENECA findings that Casodex had no effect on serum testosterone concentrations.

Effects of Casodex on Accessory Sex Organs in Adult Male Monkeys

It was important to evaluate the effect of Casodex on accessory sex organ size and plasma testosterone concentrations in monkeys, a species more closely related to man. In order to reduce the number of animals in the study, accessory sex organ sizes were assessed by a sophisticated nuclear magnetic resonance imaging procedure.

In 4 male monkeys (M nemestrina), prostate volume was reduced by about 20% after treatment for 4 weeks with 1 mg Casodex/kg and by about 30% after treatment with 5 mg Casodex/ kg for a further 2 weeks. Seminal vesicles showed more extensive shrinkage, the corresponding reduction being about 45% and 55%, respectively. Volumes recovered on withdrawal of Casodex. In an untreated animal prostate volume fell by 14% and seminal vesicle volume by 16% during the period of daily dosing by gavage.

Plasma testosterone concentrations were measured in the 4 monkeys treated with Casodex and the one treated with vehicle and subjected to periodic imaging of the prostate and seminal vesicles; marked fluctuations were seen in all the animals both during the period of treatment and afterwards but no consistent trends were apparent that could be attributed to Casodex treatment.

General Pharmacology and Toxicology of Casodex

In all studies, Casodex was well tolerated. It had no significant effects in any general pharmacology tests except in the dog where, on chronic administration, it caused a small increase in heart rate and a reduction in P-R interval at doses more than 25 times the ED_{50} value for prostate atrophy. Since there was neither impairment of cardiac function nor pathological findings when cardiac histology was examined in chronic toxicity studies, it is concluded that this idiosyncratic finding is of no toxicological consequence. This conclusion is supported by clinical observations which fail to demonstrate any effect of Casodex on cardiac function.

Casodex was shown to be a pure antiandrogen and specifically possessed neither oestrogenic nor antioestrogenic, progestational nor antiprogestational, neither glucocorticoid nor antiglucocorticoid and neither mineralocorticoid nor antimineralocorticoid activity in classical endocrine tests. Casodex also showed no androgenic activity.

Casodex has been studied in acute and chronic toxicity studies. It is well tolerated and, apart from effects related directly to its mode of action as an antiandrogen, only 2 findings require comment.

In dogs, Casodex causes a dose-related increase in heart rate and decrease in P-R interval consistent with the findings in the General Pharmacology tests. There were no pathological findings related to this physiological change and there was no impairment of cardiac function. In clinical studies [42] there were no effects on cardiac function so the change is considered to be of no relevance to man.

In toxicity studies in rats benign adenomas of the Leydig cells and thyroid were found as well as some liver tumours [43]. Leydig cell hyperplasia and adenomas are common features following alteration of the endocrine milieu in rats but are of no relevance to human exposure to the drug. This is consistent with a lack of Leydig cell hyperplasia or adenomas in testes from patients treated with Casodex [44]. The liver and thyroid tumours are related and considered to be due to the mixed function oxidase-inducing properties of Casodex in the rat. It is well recognized that agents which induce mixed function oxidases in the rat can lead to liver and thyroid tumours but that this is of no relevance to man [45-46].

Conclusions

It is concluded that Casodex:

1. Binds to rat, dog and human prostate and rat pituitary androgen receptors.
2. Inhibits growth of androgen-responsive tumours *in vitro* including one that has mutated androgen receptor and which is stimulated by flutamide and cyproterone acetate but this is, as yet, of unclear clinical significance.
3. Inhibits growth of accessory sex organs stimulated by administration of androgen in castrated rats.
4. Prevents growth of accessory sex organs in intact rats and is more potent in this respect than flutamide.
5. Inhibits growth of dog and monkey prostates.
6. Has little antiandrogenic activity at the hypothalamic-pituitary axis and, therefore, elicits only minor changes in serum luteinising hormone and testosterone concentrations in the rat, dog and monkey.
7. Is a pure antiandrogen and possesses neither androgenic nor progestational properties unlike cyproterone acetate, and has no antiprogestational, oestrogenic, antioestrogenic, glucocorticoid, mineralocorticoid or anti-gluco or mineralocorticoid properties.
8. Inhibits the rate of growth of Dunning transplantable rat prostate tumours and in this respect is as effective as surgical castration.
9. Has no significant effect in general pharmacology tests except in the dog where, on chronic administration, it causes a small increase in heart rate and a reduction in P-R interval at doses more than 25 times higher than the ED_{50} value for prostate atrophy, without impairing cardiac function.

The overall conclusion, therefore, is that Casodex is a potent, peripherally selective antiandrogen which has advantages, demonstrable in animals, over both flutamide and cyproterone acetate.

REFERENCES

1 Veterans Administration Co-operative Urological Group: Treatment and survival of patients with cancer of the prostate. Surg Gynaecol Obstet 1967 (124):1011-1017

2 Robinson MRG: Cancer of the prostate: Hormonal therapy. Clin Oncol 1982 (1):233-244

3 Neumann F and Jacobi GH: Antiandrogens in tumour therapy. Clin Oncol 1982 (1):41-65

4 Dutta AS and Furr BJA: Luteinizing hormone releasing hormone (LHRH) analogues. Ann Rep Medicinal Chemistry 1985 (20):203-214

5 Furr BJA and Milsted RAV: LH-RH analogues in cancer treatment. In: Stoll B (ed) Endocrine Management of Cancer. 2. Contemporary Therapy. Karger, Basel 1988 pp16-29

6 Debruyne FMJ, del Moral PF, Geboers ADH: LHRH analogues therapy for metastatic prostate cancer. Progress Clin Biol Res 1988 (260):27-39

7 Furr BJA and Hutchinson F: Biodegradable sustained release formulation of the LH-RH analogue 'Zoladex' for the treatment of hormone-responsive tumours. EORTC Genitourinary Group Monograph 2, Part A. Therapeutic Principles in Metastatic Prostatic Cancer. Alan R Liss, New York 1985 pp 143-153

8 Crawford D and Nabors W: Hormone therapy of advanced prostate cancer: Where we stand today. Primary Care and Cancer 1991 (11):13-20

9 Janknegt RA, Abbou CC, Bartoletti R et al: Orchiectomy and nilutamide or placebo as treatment of metastatic prostatic cancer in a multinational double-blind randomized trial. J Urol 1993 (149):77-83

10 Paisey RB, Kadow C, Bolton C, Hartog M and Gingell JC: Effects of cyproterone acetate and a long acting LHRH analogue on serum lipoproteins in patients with carcinoma of the prostate. J Royal Soc Med 1986 (79):210-211

11 Seed M, Godsland IF, Wynn V et al: The effects of cyproterone acetate and ethinyl estradiol on carbohydrate metabolism. Clin Endocrinol 1984 (21):689-699

12 Harris AL and Cantwell BMJ: Side-effects of endocrine therapies used to treat breast and prostate cancer. Clin Oncol 1985 (4):511-533

14 McFarlane JR and Tolly DA: Flutamide therapy for advanced prostate cancer: a phase II study. Br J Urol 1985 (57):172-174

15 Crawford ED, Eisenberger MA, McLeod DG, Spaulding JT, Benson R, Dorr FA, Bluemenstein DA, David MA, Goodman PJ: A controlled trial of leuprolide with and without flutamide in prostatic carcinoma. N Engl J Med 1989 (321):419-424

16 Lund F and Rasmussen F: Flutamide versus stilboestrol in the management of advanced prostate cancer. Br J Urol 1988 (61):140-142

17 Katchen B and Buxbaum S: Disposition of a new, non-steroid, antiandrogen α,α,α trifluoro-2-methyl-4-nitro-m-propionotoluidide (flutamide) in men following a single oral 200 mg dose. J Clin Endocrinol Metabol 1975 (41):371-373

18 Tremblay D, Dupont A, Meyer BJ, Pottier J: The kinetics of antiandrogens in humans. In: Murphy GP, Khoury S, Kuss R, Chatelain C and Denis L (eds): Prostate Cancer A: Research into Endocrine Treatment and Histopathology. Alan R Liss, New York 1987 pp 345-350

19 Ojasoo J: Nilutamide. Drugs of the Future 1987 (12): 763-770

20 Harnois C, Malenfant M, Dupont A, Labrie F: Ocular toxicity of Anandron in patients treated for prostate cancer. Br J Ophthalmol 1986 (70):471-473

21 Brisset JM, Bertagna L, Proulx L: Ocular toxicity of Anandron. Br J Ophthalmol 1987 (71):639

22 Furr BJA , Valcaccia B, Curry B et al: ICI 176,334: A novel non-steroidal, peripherally selective antiandrogen. J Endocrinol 1987 (113):R7-R9

23 Winneker RC, Wagner MM, Batzold FH: Studies on the mechanism of action of Win 49,596: a steroidal androgen receptor antagonist. J Steroid Biochem 1989 (33):1133-1138

24 Fuhrmann U, Bengston C, Repenthin G, Schillinger E: Stable transfection of androgen receptor and MMTV-CAT into mammalian cells: inhibition of CAT expression by antiandrogens. J Steroid Biochem 1992 (42):787-793

25 Juniewicz RE, McCarthy M, Lemp BM, Barbolt TA, Shaw C, Hollenbaugh DM, Winneker RC, Reel JR, Batzold FH: The effect of the steroidal androgen receptor antagonist, Win 49,596, on the prostate and testis of Beagle dogs. Endocrinology 1990 (126):2625-2634

26 Ayub M and Levell MJ: The effect of ketoconazole related imidazole drugs and antiandrogens on [^{3}H] R1881 binding to the prostatic androgen receptor and [^{3}H]5-dihydrotestosterone and [^{3}H]cortisol binding to plasma proteins. J Steroid Biochem 1989 (33):251-255

27 Veldscholte J, Berrevoets CA, Ris-Stalpers C, Kuiper GGJM, Jenster G, Trapman J, Brinkman AO, Mulder E: The androgen receptor in LNCaP cells contains a mutation in the ligand binding domain which affects steroid binding characteristics and response to antiandrogens. J Steroid Biochem 1992 (41):665-669

28 Freeman SN: Studies on the mechanism of action of a novel, non-steroidal antiandrogen, ICI 176,334. Ph D Thesis, University of Leeds 1988 pp 109-115

29 Veldscholte J, Berrevoets CA, Brinkmann AO, Grootegoed JA, Mulder E: Anti-androgens and the mutated androgen receptor of LNCaP cells: Differential effects on binding affinity, heat-shock protein interaction and transcription activation. Biochemistry 1992 (31):2393-2399

30 Kelly WK and Scher H: Prostate specific antigen decline after antiandrogen withdrawal: the flutamide withdrawal syndrome. J Urol 1993 (149):607-609

31 Dupont A, Gomez J-L, Cusan L, Koutsilieris M, Labrie F: Response to flutamide withdrawal in advanced prostate cancer in progression under combination therapy. J Urol 1993 (150):908-913

32 Darbre PD and King RJB: Steroid hormone regulation of cultured breast cancer cells. In: Lippman ME and Dickson R (eds) Breast Cancer and Molecular Biology. Kluwer Academic, Boston 1988 pp 307-341

33 Darbre PD and King RJB: Antiandrogen ICI 176,334 does not prevent development of androgen insen-

sitivity in S115 mouse mammary tumour cells. J Steroid Biochem 1990 (36):385-389
34 Snyder BW, Winneker RC, Batzold FJ: Endocrine profile of Win 49,596 in the rat: a novel androgen receptor antagonist. J Steroid Biochem 1989 (33): 1127-1132
35 Chandolia RK, Weinbauer GF, Behre HM, Nieschlag EL: Evaluation of a peripherally selective antiandrogen ('Casodex') as a tool for studying the relationship between testosterone and spermatogenesis in the rat. J Steroid Biochem 1991 (38):367-375
36 Chandolia RK, Weinbauer GF, Simoni M, Behre HM, Nieschlag E: Comparative effects of chronic administration of the non-steroidal antiandrogens flutamide and 'Casodex' on the reproductive system of the adult male rat. Acta Endocrinologica 1991 (125): 547-555
37 Simoni M, Weinbauer GF, Chandolia RK, Nieschlag E: Microheterogeneity of pituitary follicle-stimulating hormone in male rats: differential effects of the chronic androgen deprivation induced by castration or androgen blockade. J Mol Endocrinol 1992 (9): 175-182
38 Belchetz PE: Effects of androgens and antiandrogens on pulsatile gonadotrophin-releasing hormone secretion from the adult male rat hypothalamus in vitro. J Endocrinol 1987 (115 suppl): abstr 59
39 Freeman S N, Mainwaring WIP, Furr BJA: A possible explanation for the peripheral selectivity of a novel non-steroidal pure antiandrogen, 'Casodex' (ICI 176,334). Br J Cancer 1989 (60):664-668
40 Labrie F, Dupont A, Belanger A: Complete androgen blockade for the treatment of prostate cancer. In: De Vita VT, Hellman S, Rosenberg SA (eds) Important Advances in Oncology. Lipincott, Philadelphia 1985 pp193-200
41 Hutchinson FG and Furr BJA: Biodegradable polymers for the sustained release of peptides. Biochem Soc Transactions 1985 (13):520-523
42 Blackledge GRP: Clinical aspects of Casodex. Chapter in this Monograph
43 Eri LM and Tveter KJ: A prospective, placebo-controlled study of the antiandrogen Casodex as treatment for patients with benign prostatic hyperplasia. J Urol 1993 (150):90-94
44 Jones HB, Betton GR, Bowdler AL, McFarquahar BJ, Middleton BJ, Lunglmayr G: Pathological and morphometric assessment of testicular parameters in patients with metastatic prostate cancer following treatment with either the antiandrogen Casodex (ZM176,334) or bilateral orchiectomy. Urol Res 1994 (in press)
45 McClain RM: The significance of hepatic microsomal enzyme induction and altered thyroid function in rats: implications for thyroid neoplasia. Toxicol Pathol 1989 (17):294-306
46 McClain RM: Mouse liver tumours and microsomal enzyme-inducing drugs: experimental and clinical perspectives with phenobarbital. In: Stevenson DE, McClain RM, Popp JA, Slaga TJ, Ward JM and Pitot HC (eds) Mouse Liver Carcinogenesis: Mechanisms and Species Comparisons. Alan R Liss, New York 1990 pp 345-365

Clinical Aspects of Casodex

George R.P. Blackledge

Medical Research Department, ZENECA Pharmaceuticals, Mereside, Alderley Park, Macclesfield, Cheshire SK10 4TG, United Kingdom

Casodex* is a pure, potent, well tolerated, non-steroidal antiandrogen which is orally absorbed and has a half-life of around 7 days, allowing once-daily dosing [1]. The drug has been administered to more than 3,000 patients for periods of up to 6 years and has so far demonstrated an excellent tolerance profile permitting long-term administration. When non-steroidal antiandrogens are used as monotherapy, the pharmacological effects associated with this class of compounds, i.e., breast tenderness, gynaecomastia and hot flushes, are present in some patients. With Casodex, however, there is no evidence of lack of tolerance such as is seen in the gastrointestinal tract with flutamide, or ocular changes and alcohol intolerance as is present with nilutamide. When administered as monotherapy, Casodex has been shown in several studies to spare sexual function in the majority of sexually active males who require therapy [2].

A pure, well tolerated, non-steroidal antiandrogen can potentially be used in a number of situations; in prostate cancer these are as follows:

Advanced prostate cancer

a) As monotherapy as the primary treatment of the disease.
b) In combination with castration to provide maximal androgen blockade.
c) In combination with a 5-alpha reductase inhibitor to provide androgen blockade.
e) For the treatment of flare in association with the administration of LHRH agonists.
f) As a treatment for patients failing primary hormonal manipulation.

Early prostate cancer

a) As a debulking agent prior to radical local treatment.
b) As an adjuvant treatment following radical local therapy.

The criteria for an effective antiandrogen in these circumstances vary depending upon the concomitant therapy and also on the expectations of treatment in these different situations. The level of clinical activity of Casodex is therefore critical for deciding its precise role or roles in the management of prostate cancer.

Evidence for Clinical Activity of Casodex

In contrast with other methods of hormone manipulation for prostate cancer where changes in hormone levels are indicators of potential activity (e.g. decrease in testosterone to castrate levels with LHRH agonists), non-steroidal antiandrogens do not cause immediate changes in hormonal levels and therefore other indicators of early activity must be sought.

Retrospective analysis of studies evaluating the role of Zoladex in advanced prostate cancer had shown that Zoladex (goserelin; a medical treatment equivalent to surgical castration) resulted in a fall of at least 50% in elevated prostatic acid phosphatase (PAP) levels in two-thirds of patients. This fall in PAP was then translated into activity equivalent to castration in randomised trials. This surrogate end-

* Casodex and Zoladex are trade marks of ZENECA Limited

Table 1. Change in prostate-specific antigen (PSA) in advanced prostate cancer patients on treatment with Casodex

	Casodex dose (mg/day)					
	10	30	50	100	150	200
Number of patients	45	54	140	56	66	29
Fall in PSA at 3 months (%)	57	73	85.4	89.2	86.9	93.8

point for activity was therefore chosen for the early studies of evaluation of Casodex. A group sequential design was used for including patients in these studies and the results indicated that with 10 mg daily only 33% of patients showed a 50% or greater decrease but at 30 and 50 mg the number of patients showing a 50% or greater decrease were 53% and 83%, respectively, both fulfilling the criteria for response as set down in the protocol. In view of these findings and the excellent tolerance of Casodex, the 50 mg dose was chosen as the dose for further evaluation in both monotherapy and combination therapy [3].

Subsequent to these studies prostate specific antigen (PSA) became available and is now regarded as a more sensitive and specific tumour marker for prostate cancer [4]. More recent dose ranging studies have been carried out using fall in PSA as a surrogate endpoint. It was considered that a 50% fall in PSA would not be sufficiently large to be considered a response and therefore a 90% or greater fall in PSA has been used for these dose ranging studies. In addition to this, an assessment has been made of the number of patients whose PSA fell into the normal range during therapy. The data for PSA fall for a range of doses up to 200 mg are shown in Table 1.

These data suggest that in terms of median fall in PSA at 3 months, 50 mg does not give as good a response as 100 mg, but above 100 mg no significant differences can be detected between the doses.

In phase II studies at 50 mg and above, evidence of objective and symptomatic response was seen in studies evaluating Casodex as monotherapy [5,6]. Symptomatic response was evaluated using 3 parameters: performance status, pain score, and analgesic use. In all studies these 3 parameters improved independently in up to 70% of symptomatic patients, a clear indication of clinical activity. Objective responses have also been seen in terms of prostate size, improvement on CT scan of locally invasive disease and improvement in bone scans and skeletal X-rays [7]. From these data Casodex has clear clinical activity as a monotherapy at doses of 50 mg and above and is well tolerated [8].

Establishing a Role for Specific Indications

In order to demonstrate that Casodex has a role as monotherapy, randomised trials are necessary to demonstrate some form of benefit over standard therapy. These trials have been ongoing since 1990 and in the first instance involved a randomisation between Casodex 50 mg daily and castration in patients with D2 disease.

Three trials of similar design were conducted in North America, Europe and Scandinavia and recruited a total of over 1100 patients. In one trial, conducted in Scandinavia, there was a significant shortfall in terms of survival with Casodex when compared to castration [9]. In the other two trials, there was no significant difference in survival, although there was a trend in favour of castration [10]. This small inferiority in survival was potentially offset by quality-of-life advantages as assessed by a Qualify-of-Life Questionnaire repeated on 4 occasions following a baseline assessment prior to treatment. In particular, retention of sexual function was more likely to occur in patients receiving Casodex than castration. Symptomatic improvement was seen in both arms of the trials with roughly equal incidence. The overall conclusion from these trials was that although Casodex had shown some evidence of efficacy, it was slightly inferior in terms of time to progression and survival in comparison with castration.

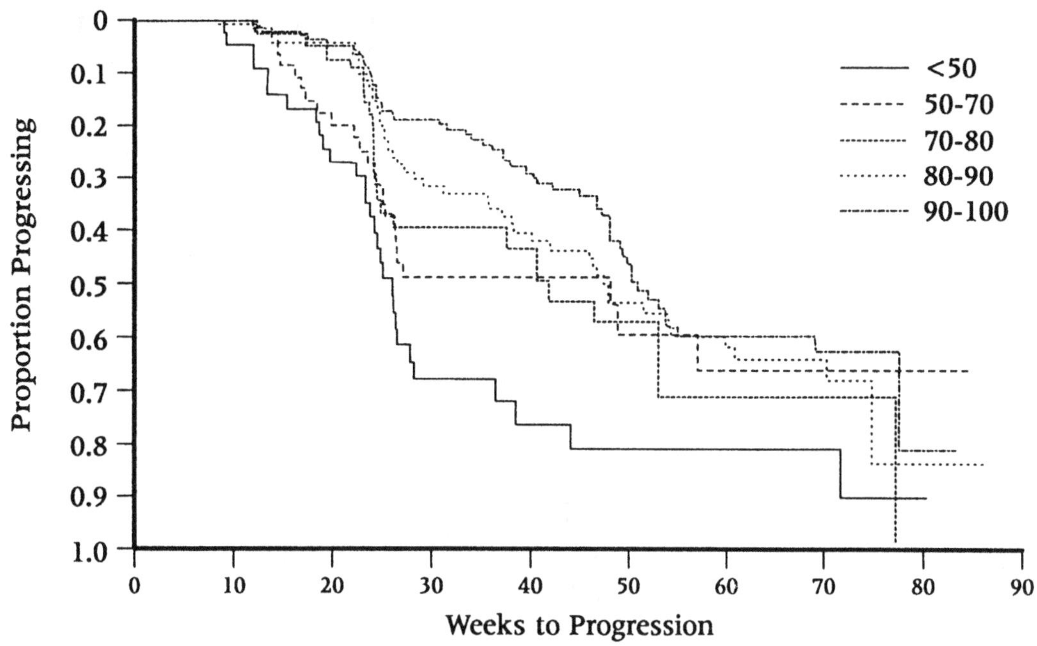

Fig. 1. Time to progression. Casodex patients by month 3 - % fall in PSA

Another interesting outcome from these studies was the observation that a decrease in PSA correlated with outcome in terms of time to progression. Figure 1 shows the correlation of PSA fall at 3 months in cohorts of patients related to time to progression. Falls in PSA early in treatment, therefore, can predict the ultimate outcome for a patient. Although this correlation is not perfect, early changes in PSA are a reasonable predictor of outcome.

Casodex 50 mg daily is also currently being evaluated in combination with castration. Since Casodex competes with androgen for occupancy of the androgen receptor, the low levels of testosterone in patients receiving medical or surgical castration should mean that Casodex is even more effective as an antiandrogen. Pharmacokinetic data suggest that a dose of 50 mg daily would be at least as effective as conventional doses of flutamide, as evidenced by the plasma levels seen with repeated dosing (Table 2), and a large multicentre trial conducted in North America comparing Casodex with flutamide with a double-blind design in associa-

Table 2. Antiandrogen levels during first week of treatment with Casodex and flutamide, with a comparison of the binding potential at the androgen receptor

	Total Casodex	Total (H) flut	Free Casodex	Free (H) flut	Casodex/(H) flut ratio of binding potential
Day 1	890	940	35.6	66	2.16
Day 2	1593	1500	63.7	105	2.43
Day 3	2348	1500	93.9	105	3.58
Day 4	2969	1500	118.8	105	4.53
Day 7	4328	1500	173.0	105	6.59

Assumes protein binding of 93% for (H) flut and 96% for Casodex and a fourfold affinity for the androgen receptor for Casodex over (H) flut

Flutamide data from Brogden and Chrisp, Drugs and Aging 1991 (1):104-115 and Radwanski et al, J Clin Pharmacol 1989 (29):554-558

Table 3. Fall in serum prostate-specific antigen (PSA) with Casodex or surgical castration allowing dose selection

	Casodex 100 mg/ day	Casodex 150 mg/ day	Castration
Mean percentage fall in PSA at 3 months	86.9	91.1	94.2
N=	63	60	28

tion with LHRH agonists has completed recruitment and is approaching the first analysis. It is anticipated that, as a component of combination therapy, Casodex 50 mg will prove at least as effective as conventional antiandrogens with an improved tolerance.

The excellent side-effect profile of Casodex, coupled with the observation of greater PSA falls with increasing dose, and evidence from pharmacokinetic studies of increased exposure with increasing dose, has meant that higher doses of Casodex could be evaluated. Two large multicentre trials were begun in 1992 with a view of comparing 2 higher doses (100 mg and 150 mg) of Casodex as monotherapy with castration. The trials had an unconventional design in that an interim analysis was carried out between the two arms of Casodex, and the one which showed the greatest PSA changes together with an acceptable all-tolerance profile, was then evaluated further against castration. The data at the time of the dose decision for PSA are shown in Table 3, where the higher dose (150 mg) was clearly superior to 100 mg.

A total of 1453 patients were recruited to these two trials and an initial analysis was carried out after a minimum of 3 months follow-up for all patients. The data from this analysis were reviewed by a Data Monitoring Committee, who strongly recommended that the follow-up on the trial continued because the data were immature with too few events having been seen in either arm. There was no evidence of any different safety profile for patients treated with 150 mg than with 50 mg and symptomatic improvement with Casodex 150 mg was at least as good as with castration. This early analysis also suggested potential quality-of-life benefits for Casodex. Further analysis of this trial when the data are more mature should be able to demonstrate the precise profile of Casodex 150 mg daily in comparison with castration and identify clearly the relevant benefits and risks of monotherapy with an antiandrogen in comparison with conventional therapy.

Definition of the Role of Casodex

Sufficient data are now being generated to be able to define the most likely roles for Casodex in the treatment of prostate cancer. It is likely that at a dose of 50 mg daily, Casodex will be an effective non-steroidal antiandrogen as part of maximal androgen blockade. Current data would suggest that this therapeutic approach is the one most likely to confirm survival benefit at the present time, especially for patients with low volume disease [11].

The role of Casodex as monotherapy in advanced prostate cancer is currently more difficult to define because of the immaturity of definitive trials. Castration is seen as highly acceptable treatment by many clinicians and patients, but others are concerned with the side-effects associated with castration and the need for either surgical intervention or parenteral administration in the case of LHRH agonists. The psychological morbidity associated with castration is also a significant factor. Assuming that there is no clinically significant difference in the conventional parameters of efficacy (time to progression and survival) for Casodex 150 mg in comparison with castration, Casodex will offer a real alternative to current conventional therapy as first-line monotherapy in advanced prostate cancer.

It is clear from current data on PSA changes with treatment for prostate cancer that falls in PSA are an extremely sensitive indicator of the effectiveness of a particular treatment. A convenient once-daily oral therapy could be monitored by measuring PSA and an early change to more conventional therapy could be considered if the PSA fall was deemed inadequate. In this way, treatment could be tailored for an individual patient offering the best benefit risk, without jeopardising the patient's ultimate outcome.

In early prostate cancer, an increasingly common presentation of the disease because of improved education and screening, Casodex could be used in several ways. The first is as a component of maximal androgen blockade to achieve cytoreduction prior to radical local treatment. Data already exist to suggest that improved surgical outcome can be achieved with pretreatment by hormone manipulation and this may translate into improvements in survival in patients with disease confined to the prostate [12].

Of potentially more importance is the role for a well-tolerated non-steroidal antiandrogen which allows retention of sexual function as an adjuvant in patients who undergo nerve-sparing radical prostatectomy for early disease and who wish to maintain quality of life including sexual function. Studies will begin during 1994 to evaluate the role of Casodex 150 mg monotherapy as an adjuvant in this context.

Conclusions

Data now exist to suggest that Casodex is an effective non-steroidal antiandrogen with a highly acceptable side-effect profile. This means that Casodex is likely to be of value at a dose of 50 mg daily in combination with castration. At higher doses it may provide an acceptable monotherapy in advanced disease, which can be monitored by changes in PSA levels. Casodex should also prove the most acceptable monotherapy for the management of early prostate cancer by hormone manipulation.

REFERENCES

1 Furr BJA, Valcaccia B, Curry B, Woodburn JR, Chesterton G, Tucker H: ICI 176,334: A novel non-steroidal, peripherally selective antiandrogen. J Endocrinol 1987 (113):R7-R9

2 Migliari R, Muscas G, Melis M, Garau M, Sorgia M, Scarpa RM, Usai E: Monitoring of penile tumescence and rigidity in patients with prostate cancer treated with 'Casodex'. Archivio Italiano di Urologia Nefrologia Andrologia 1991 (63):155-161

3 Waymont B, Blackledge G, Tyrrell CJ, Robinson MRG, Williams JL: Efficacy and safety of the non-steroidal antiandrogen 'Casodex' in early clinical trials for advanced prostate cancer. Br J Cancer 1990 (62):499

4 Oesterling JE: Prostate specific antigen: A critical assessment of the most useful tumor marker for adenocarcinoma of the prostate. J Urol 1991 (145): 907-923

5 Kasimis B, Soloway M, Robinson M, Wilding G, Lunglmayr G, Hancock A, Kennealey G, Scott M: Phase II trial of 'Casodex' in patients with advanced prostate cancer. Proc Am Soc Clin Oncol 1990 (9): 137 Abs 533. 26th Annual Meeting of the American Society of Clinical Oncology, Washington, 20-22 May 1990

6 Tyrrell CJ: 'Casodex': A pure non-steroidal anti-androgen used as monotherapy in advanced prostate cancer. Prostate 1992 (Suppl 4): 97-104. Prostate Cancer: Imaging, Management, and Screening; Proceedings of the Prostate Sessions at the 1st International Congress of the Dutch Urological Association (NVU), Rotterdam, 9-13 Oct 1991

7 Wilding G, Ahmann F, Kasimis B, Caplan R, Kennealey G: 'Casodex' efficacy and safety in study patients with advanced prostate cancer. Proc Am Soc Clin Oncol 1991 (10):182 Abs 593. 27th Annual Meeting of the American Society of Clinical Oncology, Houston, 19-21 May 1991

8 Kasimis B, Ahmann R, Schellhammer P, Smith J, Soloway M, Kennealey G, Jones J: Phase II evaluation of 'Casodex' in stage D2 prostate cancer. Proc Am Soc Clin Oncol 1992 (11):218 Abs 687. 28th Annual Meeting of the American Society of Clinical Oncology, San Diego, 17-19 May 1992

9 Iversen P, Tveter K, Varenhorst E, Study Group: Results of a Scandinavian multicentre open phase III study of 'Casodex' versus orchidectomy in the treatment of metastatic prostatic carcinoma. In: Murphy G, Khoury S, Chatelain C and Denis L (eds) Proceedings of the 3rd International Symposium on Recent Advances in Urological Cancer Diagnosis and Treatment. Paris, 17-19 Jun 1992, pp 120-125

10 Kaisary AV: Current clinical studies with a new, non-steroidal antiandrogen 'Casodex' (ICI 176,334). Clinical Developments in Prostate Cancer, 1993 (abs). Satellite Symposium held at the 2nd International Congress of the Dutch Urological Association, Amsterdam, 3 Nov 1993

11 Crawford ED, Eisenberger MA, McLeod DG, Spaulding JT, Benson R, Dorr FA, Bluemenstein DA, David MA, Goodman PJ: A controlled trial of leuprolide with and without flutamide in prostatic carcinoma. New Engl J Med 1989 (321):419-424

12 Shipley WU: A Phase III trial of androgen suppression before and during radiation therapy for locally advanced prostatic cancer: preliminary report of RTOG protocol 8610. Clinical Developments in Prostate Cancer, 1993 (abs). Satellite Symposium held at the 2nd International Congress of the Dutch Urological Association, Amsterdam, 3 Nov 1993

Pharmacodynamics and Pharmacokinetics of Nilutamide in Animal and Man

Martine Gaillard

Domaine Thérapeutique Endocrinologie, Roussel Uclaf, 102 et 111, Route de Noisy, 93230 Romainville, France

Nilutamide (RU 23908, Anandron®) is a non-steroidal antiandrogen drug; its structure is presented in Figure 1. The pharmacodynamic and pharmacokinetic profiles are reviewed in this chapter.

Pharmacodynamic Properties

Interaction with Steroid Hormone Receptors

In vitro, the relative binding affinity (RBA) of nilutamide for human steroid hormone receptors has been measured in COS cells transfected with the cDNA coding for these receptors.
Nilutamide binds specifically to the androgen receptor. After 24-hour incubation of the cytosol at 0°C, its RBA is 4% of that of testosterone and similar to that of hydroxy-flutamide and Casodex. It is about 10 times higher than the RBA for the rat prostate androgen receptor (0.3%), which binds nilutamide very weakly in comparison to other species such as mouse or dog [1].
The affinity for the other human steroid hormone receptors is undetectable; this is in contrast with steroid antiandrogens, such as cyproterone acetate, which bind to the progestin and glucocorticoid receptors. This is why nilutamide is devoid of other hormonal or antihormonal activities and is considered a "pure" antiandrogen [1,2].
In vivo, when nilutamide (10 mg/kg) was administered to castrated rats (Fig. 2), 60% to 100% of the prostate androgen binding sites were occupied during the first 16 hours due to the high plasma concentration of the compound and its slow elimination rate [3,4]. Not only the affinity for the receptor, but also the kinetics leading to a high and constant ratio of nilutamide/testosterone plasma levels are important parameters to evaluate the occupation of androgen receptors *in vivo*.

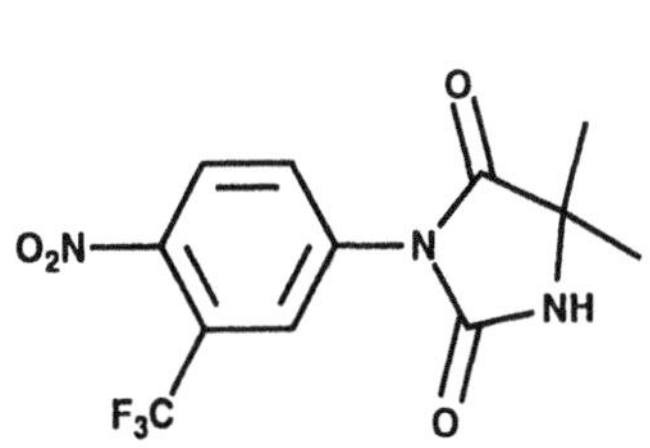

Fig. 1. Chemical structure of nilutamide

Antiandrogen Activity

In vitro:

In human breast cancer cells (T47D) transfected with the mouse-mammary tumour virus (MMTV) androgen-dependent promoter linked to the chloramphenicol acetyl-transferase (CAT) reporter gene, nilutamide produced a dose-dependent inhibition of dihydrotestosterone (DHT)-induced CAT activity [5]. A 50% inhibition of the DHT effect was obtained with a 200-fold excess of nilutamide, while a ratio of 1000 was necessary to completely abolish the DHT effect.
Nilutamide was devoid of agonist activity in this model, since it did not induce CAT activity when incubated alone at concentrations up to 10 µM.

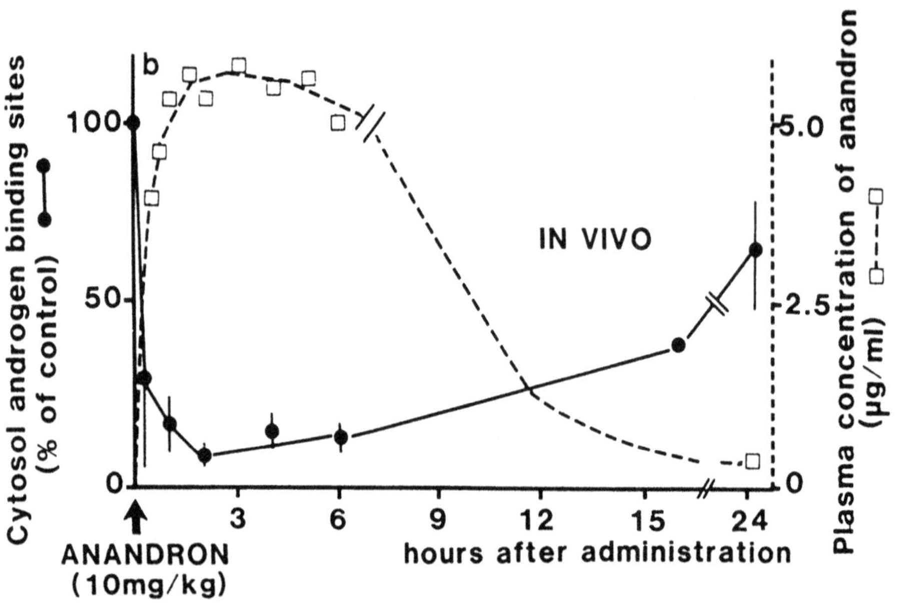

Fig. 2. Concentration of nilutamide (anandron) in plasma (□) and concentration of unoccupied androgen binding sites in prostate (●) after oral administration of 10 mg/kg of nilutamide to castrated rats [4]

In vivo:

Acute treatment with nilutamide to orchidectomised mice inhibited the testosterone-induced ornithine decarboxylase activity in the kidney 16 hours after administration [5]. A 50% inhibition was obtained at a dose of nilutamide equivalent to that of testosterone (3 mg/kg). No agonist effect was observed even at doses of 100 mg/kg, in contrast to cyproterone acetate which showed a weak agonist effect on this specific androgen-dependent enzyme activity.
Chronic treatment of castrated rats with nilutamide prevented, in a dose-dependent fashion, the increase in prostate weight induced by testosterone injected for 2 weeks [1,2] or implanted for 28 days [6]. By contrast, in intact rats even high doses of nilutamide (50 mg/kg) did not totally inhibit the trophic effects of endogenous androgens on the prostate. This is due to the occupation of pituitary androgen receptors, resulting in a blockade of the androgen-dependent negative feedback and thus in an increase in circulating testosterone which counteracts the antiandrogen effect of nilutamide at the prostate level [1,2].
The increase in testosterone is more important in the rat than in the dog. This could explain why, in addition to the much higher affinity of nilutamide for the dog androgen receptor, nilutamide has antiandrogen effects on the prostate of intact dogs with doses at least 20 times lower than in rats.
In rats castrated either by surgery (Fig. 3) or by treatment with LHRH-agonists, nilutamide was also able to inhibit the trophic effect on the prostate of adrenal androgens infused at levels equivalent to those observed in orchidectomised patients with prostate cancer [4].

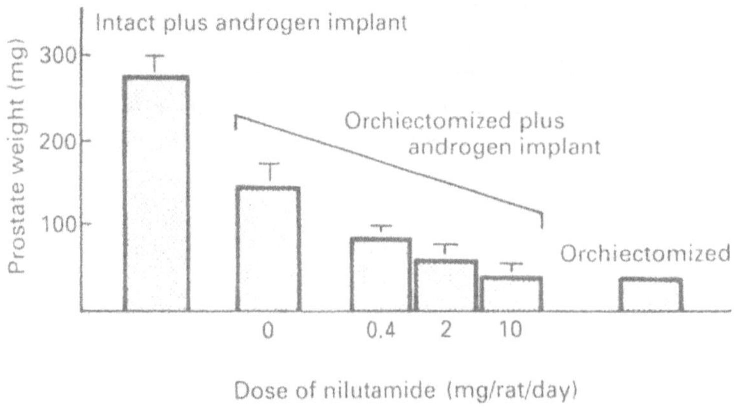

Fig. 3. Inhibition by nilutamide of the trophic effect on prostate of adrenal androgens infused by minipumps ("androgen implant") for 15 days in rats in order to have plasma levels equivalent to those of humans. A group of orchidectomised rats with no adrenal androgen supplementation was taken as total androgen-deprived controls [4]

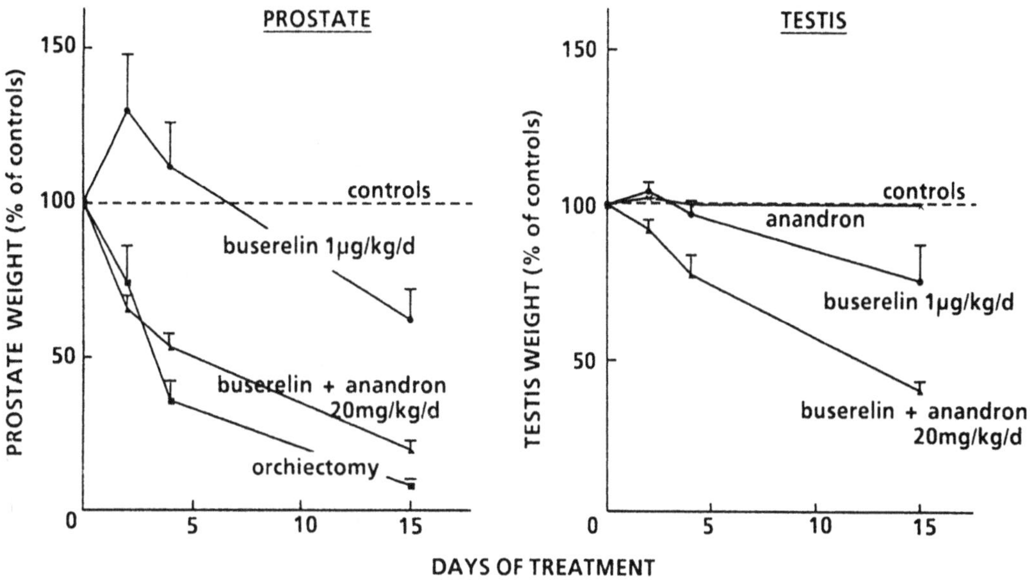

Fig. 4. Inhibition by nilutamide of the initial effect of a buserelin treatment in rat on prostate and testis weight. Intact rats received daily for 2, 4 or 15 days, injections of buserelin alone or combined with oral administration of nilutamide (anandron). Control intact rats and orchidectomised rats received solvent only. Prostates and testes were weighed [7]

When intact rats were given daily s.c. injections of the LHRH-agonist buserelin, the weight of the prostate transiently increased as a result of the transient increase in testosterone due to the initial agonist effect of the analogue, and only began to decrease after 6 to 7 days (Fig. 4). Concomitant treatment with nilutamide (20 mg/kg/day) prevented this initial "flare" effect of buserelin [1,5]. Moreover, testis atrophy induced by buserelin treatment was more pronounced when nilutamide was administered with buserelin, while nilutamide alone had no effect on testis weight (Fig. 4).

This was also true when rats were treated for longer periods with implants of buserelin (Fig. 5). Moreover, the level of plasma testosterone that was not totally suppressed in the rat by buserelin injections [7] or implants (Fig. 5), was reduced to levels seen in orchidectomised animals by the combination treatment of buserelin with nilutamide [7,8]. Nilutamide treatment alone increased plasma testosterone level.

Nilutamide thus seems to potentiate the "castrating" effect of the LHRH-agonist on the testis, in addition to the blockade exerted directly at the prostate androgen receptor level against residual androgens.

Activity in Androgen-Dependent Tumour Cell Lines

In vitro, in addition to the antiandrogen activity observed in T47D cells (see above), antiandrogen effects of nilutamide were also observed on the proliferation of AXC/SShT rat prostate cancer cell line, whether androgens promoted or inhibited cell growth [9]. At high concentrations (>10 µM), nilutamide displayed cytotoxic activity in these cells even in the absence of testosterone [9]. We observed similar antiproliferative effects of high concentrations of nilutamide on breast cancer cell lines (MCF7 and T 47D).

In vivo, nilutamide was also shown to reduce the incidence and development of the androgen-dependent Shionogi tumour (SC 115) in mice [1,5] and Dunning prostatic tumour in rats [10].

Inhibition of Androgen Synthesis

In addition to its antiandrogen activity at the receptor level, nilutamide may also inhibit the synthesis of androgens. An *in vitro* study using microsomes from rat testis [11] demonstrated

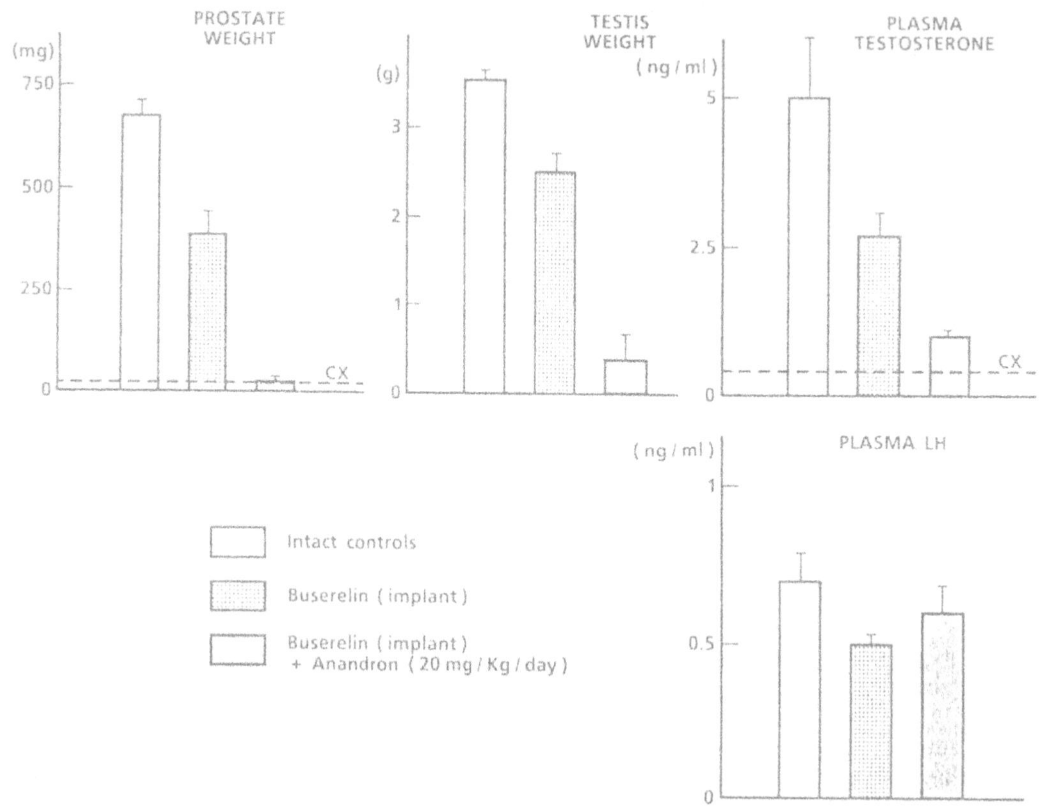

Fig. 5. Potentiation by nilutamide of the "castrating" effect of buserelin implanted for 6 weeks in intact male rats. Intact male rats were implanted with a "depot" form of buserelin (gift of Dr J. Sandow, Hoechst, Germany) and treated with solvent or nilutamide (anandron, 20 mg/kg/day) orally for 6 weeks. A group of intact rats and a group of castrated rats were taken as controls. Prostates and testes were weighed and plasma LH and testosterone were measured by radioimmunoassay.

that nilutamide at concentrations over 50 μM inhibited the activity of 17 α hydroxylase and 17,20 lyase activity, as did hydroxyflutamide and cyproterone acetate.

Pharmacokinetic Properties

Pharmacokinetics in Animals

In the rat, the plasma kinetics were studied using ^{14}C-labeled nilutamide, which was administered either intravenously (10 mg/kg) or orally [3]. Bioavailability by oral route was complete. The absorption half-life was 0.34 hour. The majority of the plasma radioactivity was unchanged nilutamide up to 6 hours, $t_{1/2}$ was 7 hours. By 72 hours, 90% was in the form of metabolites.

In the dog, the pharmacokinetic parameters for the unchanged drug were similar to those in the rat [3].

Pharmacokinetics in Men

The pharmacokinetics of nilutamide were studied in 12 healthy human volunteers [3,12]. After administration of a single oral dose of 100, 200 or 300 mg, separated by a 2-week interval according to a randomised cross-over design, the drug plasma level was dose dependent and declined in a log-linear fashion with time after a short distribution phase. The three doses had similar half-lives (around 45 hours).

In 12 patients with metastatic prostate cancer, the pharmacokinetics of nilutamide were studied after oral administration of a single dose of ^{14}C nilutamide, followed 4 or 8 days later by treatment with unlabeled nilutamide (150 mg b.i.d.) which continued for 2 to 7 weeks [3,13]. The

Table 1. Kinetic parameters in 12 patients with metastatic prostate cancer

	Total radioactivity	Unchanged nilutamide
C_{max} (mg/l)	1.29 ± 0.08	0.9 ± 0.07
T_{max} (h)	5.8 ± 1.1	2.8 ± 0.3
AUC (mg/l/h	136 ± 7	38.6 ± 2.7
$t_{1/2}$ (h)	86.9 ± 7.8	56.3 ± 5.4

pharmacokinetic parameters after the single radioactive dose are summarised in Table 1. The plasma elimination half-life of nilutamide was longer than in volunteers (mean = 56 h). Total radioactivity has a longer plasma half-life than the drug alone, suggesting that clearance of the metabolites is slower that the non-metabolised compound. The plateau level of nilutamide (steady state) was obtained after about 14 days of repeated administration of the drug (150 mg b.i.d.) and did not depend upon intervals between doses.
Excretion of radioactivity in the faeces was negligible (1.4, 1.6 and 7% of total dose recovered after 4 to 5 days in 3 patients). Recovery in the urine was high (61.6% total radioactivity recovered at 5 days, only 0.8% as unchanged drug). This indicates that the absorption of nilutamide through the gastrointestinal tract is virtually complete.
Nilutamide concentrations were recorded over a 12-month period in patients participating in a multicentre clinical trial [12] (Table 2). The plasma concentrations recorded with the 300 mg dose were twice as high as those recorded with the 150 mg dose, indicating that the kinetics are linear. No significant changes were found in the plasma levels during the 12 months of administration.

Table 2. Mean plasma nilutamide concentrations (mg/l) during treatment of patients

Month	150 mg/day	300 mg/day
1	3.4 ± 1.1 (n=26)	7.2 ± 3.6 (n=33)
3	3.6 ± 1.2 (n=32)	7.3 ± 3.9 (n=31)
6	3.7 ± 1.7 (n=28)	7.4 ± 2.7 (n=27)
12	3.8 ± 0.9 (n=14)	7.0 ± 2.7 (n=12)

Metabolism

The metabolism of nilutamide in animals and humans is intensive [3,14]. The site of primary attack is the nitro group attached to the benzene ring which is reduced. The antiandrogen activity of the principal metabolites is weak or undetectable, suggesting that they probably contribute little to the overall activity of nilutamide.

Clinical Pharmacology

Study of the Antiandrogenic Effects of Nilutamide in Healthy Males

In order to study the physiological effects of nilutamide on the endocrine system of healthy males, nilutamide (150 mg b.i.d.) was given orally for 8 weeks to 15 male subjects who presented for male to female gender transformation. None of the subjects had been using hormonal drugs previously [15,16].
As expected, the interruption of the negative feedback of androgens led to an increase in plasma LH (but not FSH) which resulted in stimulation of testicular steroidogenesis. Testosterone, androstenedione, DHEA, DHEAs, oestrone and oestradiol levels rose, the major part of the increase occurring within 4 to 6 weeks, after which no further changes occurred. Prolactin and SBP increased probably as a result of the rise in oestradiol. The LHRH-stimulated LH levels rose progressively during the first 6 weeks and a new equilibrium was reached within 4 weeks. By contrast, the LHRH-stimulated FSH tended to be reduced, probably due to oestradiol, which selectively inhibits FSH in comparison to LH.
Both the amount and the weight of sexual hair displayed a downward trend reflecting the antiandrogen activity of Anandron [16].

Prevention of the Transient Adverse Effects of a LHRH Agonist Buserelin in Patients with Metastatic Prostate Carcinoma

A double-blind placebo-controlled study was conducted to evaluate the efficacy of nilutamide in inhibiting the adverse effects observed at the start of treatment of prostatic cancer with an LHRH agonist [17].

Thirty-six men with disseminated prostatic cancer and elevated plasma levels of prostatic acid phosphatase (PAP) were randomly assigned to two groups of treatment: buserelin (500 µg/day s.c.) and nilutamide (300 mg daily orally), and buserelin and placebo. Bone pain was assessed by a visual analogue scale and by a calculation of the consumption of analgesics, and plasma was collected before and during treatment.

Bone pain appeared or worsened in 12 of the 19 men in the buserelin + placebo group while in only 5 of the 17 men in the buserelin + nilutamide group. Median levels of PSA decreased from day 8 in the buserelin + placebo group while they decreased immediately in the combination with nilutamide group (Fig. 6). The median concentration of plasma PAP increased transiently and then decreased on day 14 in the buserelin + placebo group while it decreased almost immediately in the LHRH + nilutamide group.

Testosterone levels similarly increased (doubled) at the start of the treatment in the two groups (Fig. 6), but thereafter the median time to obtain levels corresponding to that obtained after orchidectomy (0.20 ng/ml) was significantly shorter in the buserelin + anandron-treated group (22 days) than in the buserelin + placebo-treated group (more than 29 days). Testosterone levels were different between the two groups from day 11. Androstenedione levels were also significantly decreased from day 6 in the anandron-treated group.

This study shows that nilutamide (300 mg/day) not only is able to prevent the adverse consequences ("flare") of the LHRH agonist-induced transient rise in plasma testosterone levels in men with metastatic prostate cancer, but might also potentiate or accelerate the castrating effect of buserelin.

Dose Determination Studies

An open study in patients with metastatic prostate cancer treated for 7 days with 50, 100, 300 or 600 mg/day of nilutamide demonstrated the satisfactory safety of doses up to 300 mg/day and an antiandrogenic activity, reflected by an increase in plasma LH, in most patients receiving 100, 300 and 600 mg/kg.

Thereafter, due to concerns of increased plasma testosterone concentrations which might neutralise the beneficial antiandrogen effect of the drug at the level of the cancer cell, most clinical studies were performed in orchidectomised or LHRH agonist-treated patients.

The determination of the optimal dose regimen was thus made in orchidectomised patients. A double-blind study was performed to compare the efficacy and safety of the highest safe dose (300 mg/day) and half of this dose and placebo. Metastatic prostate cancer patients not treated previously were surgically castrated and randomly assigned to receive nilutamide 300 mg/day (62 patients) or 150 mg/day (66 patients) or placebo (63 patients) for 24 months or until disease progression.

The main efficacy criterion was objective response to treatment (National Prostate Cancer Project (NPCP) criteria) and the secondary criteria were modifications of clinical disease parameters (pain, performance status, urinary obstruction) and laboratory parameters (prostatic acid phosphatase and alkaline phosphatase).

This study showed a quite similar efficacy of the two doses on response rate and disease criteria, and a lower frequency of the most frequent adverse events with the lower dose.

These results, together with pharmacokinetic findings showing that an effective plasma level was reached earlier with 300 mg/day, led to the recommendation for the dosage regimen of nilutamide combined with castration of a loading dose of 300 mg once daily followed by 150 mg once daily after one month or earlier if intolerance occurred. Although steady state of nilutamide is reached after 2 weeks, month 1 was chosen for dose reduction for practical considerations: the first visit during treatment was after 1 month and furthermore, during treatment with LHRH agonists, castration level of testosterone is reached within 1 month.

Discussion

By preventing their binding to the androgen receptor level, nilutamide blocks the effect of testicular and adrenal androgens on their different target cells. The antiandrogen activity and the absence of agonist effects of nilutamide have been extensively demonstrated in normal as well as tumoral tissues in different species including man.

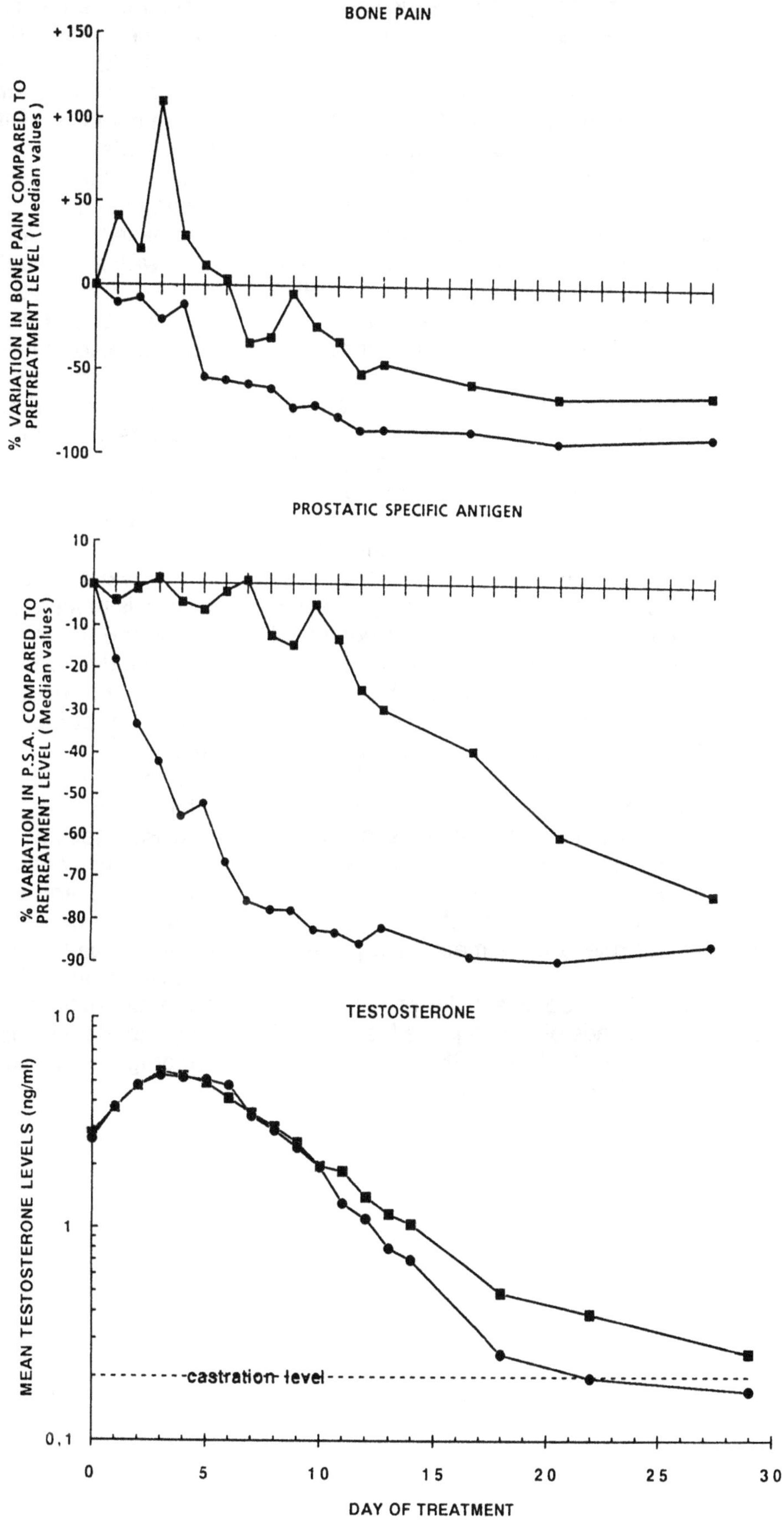

Fig. 6. Inhibition of "flare" effect of initial rise in testosterone induced by buserelin treatment in metastatic prostate cancer patients. Median change in bone pain and prostate specific antigen (PSA) and mean testosterone concentrations in patients treated either with buserelin (500 mg/day sc) and nilutamide (300 mg/day oral) (●) or with buserelin and placebo (■) [17]

In addition to its antiandrogenic effect at the receptor, an *in vitro* study on rat testicular microsomes suggests that nilutamide, at concentrations (50 µM) that could be reached in adrenal tissue *in vivo*, may also inhibit the activity of enzymes implicated in the synthesis of androgens, in particular those of adrenal origin [11]. Evidence for such a role of nilutamide is provided by clinical studies in patients with prostate cancer castrated either by surgery [18] or by LHRH agonists [17,19], in whom the plasma concentrations of androstenedione or DHEA were reduced during nilutamide treatment. However, plasma cortisol levels remained unchanged.

Finally, the antiproliferative effect observed with nilutamide at high concentrations, even in cells cultured in the absence of androgens [9], points at the possibility that nilutamide may have a direct cytotoxic effect on the tumour. This hypothesis is contradicted by the observation in human prostatic cancer LNCaP cell lines in culture, that nilutamide, like hydroxyflutamide, cyproterone acetate and also oestradiol and progesterone, but not Casodex, has androgen-like effects on growth [20] but also on the activation of an androgen-dependent transfected reporter gene [21]. However, a mutation of the androgen receptor of the LNCaP cells in the steroid binding region is responsible for the agonist activity of the antiandrogens in this cell line [21], and since no such mutation has been found in samples of human prostate so far [22, 23], observations made in LNCaP cells are probably not relevant for metastatic prostate cancer.

The pure antiandrogen activity of nilutamide leads to a blockade of the negative feedback of testosterone, increasing LHRH activity at the pituitary and thus LH and testosterone secretion in animals [2] and in men [15]. In men, testosterone levels plateau after only a 2-fold increase, but in order to obtain maximum androgen blockade nilutamide was mostly given in surgically or chemically castrated patients. When combined with LHRH agonist treatment, nilutamide not only inhibits adrenal androgen action but also the "flare" effect at the start of treatment [1,17]. Furthermore, the testosterone decrease triggered by the LHRH agonist buserelin was accentuated by adding nilutamide in rats [7] and in patients [17]. Nilutamide may increase LHRH-A activity not only at the pituitary but also at the testis where LHRH receptors that might regulate testosterone secretion have been described, at least in the rat [24].

The kinetics of nilutamide is an additional advantage of the compound [3]. Nilutamide is fully absorbed by the oral route and does not need to be transformed into an active metabolite. The time to reach steady-state plasma levels and thus maximum therapeutic activity, about 2 weeks, is related to the long half-life of the compound (56 hours in patients), but it was shown in the study in which patients were treated for 1 month with buserelin and nilutamide 300 mg/day [17] that from the very beginning of treatment nilutamide was able to counteract the initially doubled testosterone as reflected by the inhibition of the "disease flare" on pain, PAP and PSA levels. Once the steady state was reached, nilutamide plasma concentrations are very stable and should produce a sustained receptor blockade. Finally, the long plasma elimination half-life of nilutamide offers the convenience of once-daily dosage and the subsequent benefits for compliance. This is particularly important in the elderly population in whom the drug is most likely to be used.

REFERENCES

1 Moguilewsky M, Cotard M, Proulx L, Tournemine C and Raynaud JP: What is an antiandrogen and what is the physiological and pharmacological rationale for combined "castration + antiandrogen" therapy. In: Murphy G, Khoury S, Küss R, Chatelain C and Denis L (eds) Prostate Cancer. Part A: Research, Endocrine Treatment and Histopathology. Progress in Clinical and Biological Research. AR Liss, New York 1987 pp 315-340

2 Raynaud JP, Bonne C, Moguilewsky M, Lefebvre FA, Belanger A and Labrie F: The pure antiandrogen RU 23908 (Anandron), a candidate of choice for the combined antihormonal treatment of prostatic cancer: a review. Prostate 1984 (5):299-311

3 Creaven PJ, Pendyala L and Tremblay D: Pharmacokinetics and metabolism of nilutamide. Urology 1991 (37 suppl):13-19

4 Moguilewsky M, Fiet J, Tournemine C, Raynaud JP: Pharmacology of antiandrogen, Anandron, used as an adjuvant in the treatment of prostate cancer. J Steroid Biochem 1986 (24):139-146

5 Gaillard-Moguilewsky M: Pharmacology and antiandrogens and value of combining androgen suppression with antiandrogen therapy. Urology 1991 (37 suppl):5-12

6 Dhar JD and Setty BS: Effect of a nonsteroidal antiandrogen, Anandron, on the reproductive system and fertility in male rats. Contraception 1990 (42): 121-138

7 Moguilewsky M and Tournemine C: The antiandrogen Anandron potentiates the castrating effect of the LH-RH agonist buserelin in the rat. Am J Clin Oncol 1988 (11 suppl 2):S148-S151

8 Lamberts SWJ, Uitterlinden P and DeJong FM: Rat prostatic weight regression in reaction to ketoconazole, cyproterone acetate and RU23908 as adjuncts to a depot formulation of gonadotropin releasing hormone analogue. Cancer Res 1988 (48): 6063-6068

9 Huot RI and Shain SA: Differential androgen modulation of AXC/SSh rat prostate cancer cell proliferation in vitro and its antagonism by antiandrogen. Cancer Res 1986 (46):3775-3781

10 Proulx L and Labrie F: Prostate 1984 (5):370 (abstr)

11 Ayub M and Levell MJ: Inhibition of rat testicular 17-hydroxylase and 17,20-lyase activities by antiandrogens (flutamide, hydroxyflutamide, RU 23908, cyproterone acetate) in vitro. J Steroid Biochem 1987 (28):43-47

12 Tremblay D, Dupront A, Meyer BH and Pottier J: The kinetics of anti-androgens in humans. In: Murphy G, Khoury S, Küss R, Chatelain C and Denis L (eds) Prostate Cancer. Part A: Research, Endocrine Treatment and Histopathology. Progress in Clinical and Biological Research. AR Liss, New York 1987 pp 341-350

13 Pendyala L, Creaven PJ, Huben R, Tremblay D and Bertagna C: Pharmacokinetics of Anandron in patients with advanced carcinoma of the prostate. Cancer Chemother Pharmacol 1988 (22):69-76

14 Raynaud JP, Moguilewsky M, Tournemine C, Pottier J, Coussedière D et al: Pharmacology and clinical studies with RU 23908 (Anandron). In: EORTC Genitourinary Group Monograph II. Part A: Therapeutic Principles in Metastatic Prostatic Cancer. AR Liss, New York 1985 pp 99-120

15 Gooren L, Soinder T, Spijkstra JJ, Van Kessel H, Smals A et al: Sex steroids and pulsatile luteinizing hormone release in men. Studies in estrogen-treated agonadal subjects and eugonadal subjects treated with a novel nonsteroidal antiandrogen. J Clin Endocrinol Metab 1987 (64):763-770

16 Asscheman H, Gooren LJG and Peereboom-Wynia JDR: Reduction in undesired sexual hair growth with Anandron in male-to-female transexuals - experiences with a novel androgen receptor blocker. Clin Exper Dermatol 1989 (14):361-363

17 Kuhn JM, Billebaud T, Navratil H, Moulonguet A, Fiet J et al: Prevention of the transient adverse effects of a gonadotrophin-releasing hormone analogue (buserelin) in metastatic prostatic carcinoma by administration of an antiandrogen (nilutamide). N Engl J Med 1989 (321):413-418

18 Fiet J, Villette JM, Brisset JM, Hucher M, Husson JM et al: Plasma hormone levels before and after orchiectomy in prostate cancer patients and action of a non-steroid antiandrogen anandron. In: Khoury S et al (eds) Urology: Prostate Cancer. FIIS et RGP, Boissy-le-Cutté 1990 pp 329-337

19 Belanger A, Dupont A, Labrie F: Inhibition of basal and adrenocorticotropin-stimulated plasma levels of adrenal androgens after treatment with an antiandrogen in castrated patients with prostatic cancer. J Clin Endocrinol Metab 1984 (59):422-426

20 Wilding G, Chen M, Gelmann EP: Aberrant response in vitro of hormone-responsive prostate cancer cells to antiandrogens. Prostate 1989 (14):103-115

21 Veldscholte J, Berevoets CA, Brinkmann AO, Grootegoed JA, Mulder E: Anti-androgens and the mutated androgen receptor of LNCaP cells: differential effects on binding affinity, heat-shock protein interaction and transcription activation. Biochemistry 1992 (31):2392-2399

22 Culig Z, Klocker H, Eberle J, Kaspar F, Hobisch A, Cronauer MV and Bartsch G : DNA sequence of the androgen receptor in prostatic tumor cell lines and tissue specimens assessed by means of the polymerase chain reaction. Prostate 1993 (22):11-22

23 Newmark JR, Hardy DO, Tonb DC, Carter BS, Epstein JI, Isaacs WB, Brown TR and Barrack ER: Androgen receptor gene mutations in human prostate cancer. Proc Natl Acad Sci USA 1992 (89): 6319-6323

24 Sharpe RM, Fraser HM: Leydig cell receptors for luteinizing hormone and its agonists and their modulation by administration or deprivation of the releasing hormone. Biochem Biophys Res Commun 1980 (95):256-262

A Review of the Clinical Studies with Nilutamide

Charles Mahler

Department of Endocrinology, A.Z. Middelheim, Lindendreef 1, 2020 Antwerp, Belgium

The currently available antiandrogens are of two types: steroidal and non-steroidal (pure). The first group not only interferes with the cellular androgen receptor but also displays some progestagen-like antigonadotrophic activity. Cyproterone acetate (CPA) is the best known of these. The second group, the pure antiandrogens, displaces T from the androgen receptor, lifting the negative feedback of T to the hypothalamic pituitary level; this leads to a compensatory rise of LH resulting in an increase in T production and secretion. Although there has been concern that this rise in T levels might override the blocking effects of pure antiandrogens, several reports have shown this not to be true.

In this chapter we will review and discuss the effects, therapeutic indications and side-effects of nilutamide (Anandron®).

Due to its effect on the hypothalamic-pituitary gonadal axis the drug has been mainly developed in combination with castration, either surgical or medical, in stage D_2 prostate cancer patients. The usual daily dose is 300 mg for 1 month, starting simultaneously with the castration procedure, followed by 150 mg thereafter. Its 56-hour half-life and kinetic properties allow a once-daily administration which is generally well tolerated and improves compliance in these mostly elderly patients.

Therapeutic Efficacy in Prostate Cancer

Nilutamide as Monotherapy

The activity of nilutamide as a single agent was evaluated in an open multicentre study in 44 patients with metastatic carcinoma of the prostate. This group included 26 previously untreated patients and 18 patients progressing after failure of first-line hormonal manipulation.

Objective partial responses were observed in 38.5% and 5.5%, respectively, of the two subgroups. Median progression-free survival and overall survival were 9 and 23 months, respectively, in the previously untreated patients, and 6 and 17 months in the other subgroup.

The most frequent side-effects were delayed visual adaptation to darkness, slight nausea and alcohol intolerance.

Half of the patients who had reported a normal sexual activity before therapy initiation, claimed preservation of libido and sexual potency during the treatment .

The authors conclude that single non-steroidal antiandrogen therapy deserves comparison to the more conventional modalities of endocrine treatment, especially if the patient is eager to maintain his sexual potency [1,2]. Nevertheless, the small number of patients and the open label design of the trial do not allow any definitive conclusion.

Nilutamide in Combination Therapy: Maximal Androgen Blockade

Nilutamide in combination with orchidectomy

Placebo-controlled studies are the best way to assess the efficacy of combined therapy; however, the difficulty in this design is that an equally effective treatment is part of both arms of compared modalities and that such studies may require large numbers of patients to make sure a difference exists (or not).

Table 1. Overview of placebo-controlled studies of Anandron with orchidectomy

Author	Ref.	Year	No. pts. entered	No. pts. eligible
Brisset et al.	[28]	1990	122	97
Brisset et al.	[28]	1990	191	159
Beland et al.	[15]	1991	208	194
Namer et al.	[14]	1990	151	122
Du Plessis	[29]	1990	11	11
Knönagel et al	[30]	1989	51	50
Janknegt et al.	[16]	1993	457	423
TOTAL			1191	1056

Recently a meta-analysis of all double-blind long-term randomised studies comparing orchidectomy plus Anandron versus orchidectomy plus placebo in previously untreated patients with advanced prostate cancer was completed by Bertagna et al. [3]. Seven trials were analyzed, all of similar design and using the NPCP criteria, including 1191 patients among whom 1056 eligible (Table 1).

After 6 months pain improvement was significantly better in the Anandron-treated group (48% versus 34%) (Table 2). As far as performance status and micturition-related problems were concerned the difference between both groups was slightly in favour of the Anandron group.

Among patients with abnormal pretreatment values of PAP there were significantly more normalizations within 6 months; 66% of the Anandron patients versus 53% of the placebo group (Table 3). Similarly, normalization of alkaline phosphatase was significantly more frequent, in 44% and 27%, respectively (Table 4). The percentage of regressions (complete or partial) was 50% in the Anandron group against 33% in the patients on placebo ($p < 0.001$) (Table 5). Disease progression rate within 6 months after orchidectomy was significantly lower among the Anandron recipients (21% versus 33%, $p = 0.001$).

With regard to long-term endpoints this analysis shows that the combination with nilutamide results in a 16% reduction in the risk of progression and a 10% reduction in the risk of death at any time. Although the difference is statistically significant for progression ($p = 0.050$) and not for survival, there is a trend in survival that is equatable with the difference in progression.

Table 2. Overview of placebo-controlled studies of Anandron with orchidectomy

			Metastatic pain improvement					
			Orchidectomy + Placebo			Orchidectomy + Anandron		
Author	Ref.	Year	No. pts.	Improved	Worsened	No. pts.	Improved	Worsened
Brisset et al.	[28]	1990	43	26%	7%	40	40%	5%
Brisset et al.	[28]	1990	45	22%	16%	92	42%	5%
Beland et al.	[15]	1991	72	33%	13%	81	54%	4%
Namer et al.	[14]	1990	55	38%	11%	43	37%	7%
Knönagel et al.	[30]	1989	18	56%	6%	19	32%	5%
Janknegt et al.	[16]	1993	167	37%	17%	164	54%	2%
TOTAL			400	34%	14%	439	48%	8%

$p < 0.001$

Table 3. Overview of placebo-controlled studies of Anandron with orchidectomy

		Number and percentage of normalizations of PAP at 6 months			
		Orchidectomy + Placebo		Orchidectomy + Anandron	
Author	Ref.	No. pts.	Normalization	No. pts.	Improved
Brisset et al.	[28]	24	12 = 50%	25	13 = 52%
Brisset et al.	[28]	22	12 = 50%	54	37 = 69%
Beland et al.	[15]	61	25 = 57%	61	42 = 69%
Namer et al	[14]	40	20 = 50%	29	20 = 69%
Knönagel et al.	[30]	16	6 = 37%	14	10 = 71%
Janknegt et al.	[16]	122	66 = 54%	125	81 = 65%
TOTAL		285	151 = 53%	308	203 = 66%

$p = 0.002$

Table 4. Overview of placebo-controlled studies of Anandron with orchidectomy

		Number and percentage of normalizations of ALP at 6 months			
		Orchidectomy + Placebo		Orchidectomy + Anandron	
Author	Ref.	No. pts.	Normalization	No. pts.	Improved
Brisset et al.	[28]	20	6 = 30%	15	7 = 47%
Brisset et al.	[28]	15	4 = 27%	32	16 = 50%
Beland et al.	[15]	53	10 = 19%	63	30 = 48%
Namer et al	[14]	25	10 = 40%	12	5 = 42%
Knönagel et al.	[30]	12	2 = 17%	11	3 = 27%
Janknegt et al.	[16]	106	30 = 28%	100	41 = 41%
TOTAL		231	62 = 27%	233	102 = 44%

$p < 0.001$

Table 5. Overview of placebo-controlled studies of Anandron with orchidectomy

Best response to treatment*: Number and percentage of complete and partial responses					
		Orchidectomy + Placebo		Orchidectomy + Anandron	
Author	Ref.	No. pts.	CR + PR	No. pts.	CR + PR
Brisset et al.	[28]	46	26 = 57%	41	24 = 59%
Brisset et al.	[28]	47	20 = 43%	95	58 = 61%
Beland et al.	[15]	90	18 = 20%	87	39 = 45%
Namer et al.	[14]	59	31 = 53%	45	31 = 69%
Knönagel et al.	[30]	21	6 = 29%	21	10 = 48%
Janknegt et al.	[16]	182	44 = 24%	175	72 = 41%
TOTAL		445	145 = 33%	464	234 = 50%

$p < 0.001$
* NPCP criteria

In this meta-analysis the two studies [15,16] which included the larger numbers of patients were designed with time to progression as the main endpoint. Time to objective progression was significantly longer in the Anandron group in both studies and subjective progression assessed in the trial published by Janknegt [15] was also significantly prolonged by the addition of nilutamide.

An open study performed by Akaza [4] and another randomised multicentre trial published by Le Duc [5], which were not included in the meta-analysis due to different design and duration, yielded results consistent with those reported by the meta-analysis.

Nilutamide in combination with GnRH analogues

Randomised and double-blind trials have evaluated the efficacy of the combination of Anandron and GnRH analogues (buserelin, leuprolide). Several of these studies provide substantial support to the role of the antiandrogen in preventing disease flare [6-9]. Although the amazing initial response rate of 97% reported by Labrie [6] in uncontrolled open studies could not be confirmed by subsequent randomised studies, there is no doubt that objective and subjective response rates were always higher in the cohorts of patients treated with the combination therapy, even if total survival was not considerably improved [8,10-11].

In a large (411 patients) double-blind randomised study Crawford et al. compared the effects of combination therapy (leuprolide plus Anandron) with leuprolide plus placebo [12]. Complete or partial responses were achieved in 53% of the maximal androgen withdrawal group against 41% of the placebo group ($p = 0.02$). Pain and performance status improvements were also significantly greater in the combination group. In patients with elevated prostate-specific antigen (PSA) at entry, PSA normalization occurred at month 1 in 36% in the combination group versus 13% in the placebo group ($p < 0.001$).

Alkaline phosphatase (ALP) normalized at months 3, 6 and 12 in 36% vs 13%, 56% vs 31% and 53% vs 25% of the patients. This normalization paralleled the significant improvement observed on bone scans.

The difference in median time to progression (2.1 months in favour of the Anandron group), however, was not statistically significant at the time of publication of the trial and maturation of the study is required.

From these observations it seems clear that there is a therapeutic advantage in using combination therapy with Anandron over medical castration with GnRH analogues alone.

The Effect of Nilutamide on the Prostatic Tumour Markers

Several trials comparing nilutamide versus placebo following orchidectomy or medical castration have measured changes in the levels of ALP, PSA and/or prostatic acid phosphatase (PAP). In each study there was an improvement in one or both markers when patients were given nilutamide [9,12-16].

Bertagna in the meta-analysis of 7 double-blind randomised trials comparing nilutamide and orchidectomy versus placebo and orchidectomy reported normalization of PAP and ALP values in 66% of nilutamide versus 53% of placebo receivers among those patients who had abnormal pretreatment levels [3].

Findings in two large trials comparing nilutamide versus placebo with orchidectomy or with leuprolide where PSA was prospectively and centrally assayed in 494 patients at each study time point, showed that with 98% of patients having abnormal baseline levels, normalization of PSA levels to pretreatment values occurred at a significantly higher rate in the nilutamide group. Both conclude that normalization at months 3 and 6 is the earliest and most highly correlated predictor of long-term survival and outcome. In both studies PSA nadir was reached within 3 months and normalization occurred in a significantly greater percentage of patients in the nilutamide groups than in the control groups, 57% vs 28% in the orchidectomy study and 78% vs 59% in the leuprolide trial [16-18].

Dosage and Administration

Dose ranging studies and time of initiation of drug administration have shown that 300 mg given orally as a single daily dose during the first month and 150 mg thereafter are effective. The long half-life of around 55 hours allows

single daily dosage which is in general well tolerated and improves compliance in these prevailingly elderly patients.
When medical castration is induced by GnRH agonists, flare prevention requires the simultaneous administration of the drug in order to block and limit the possible adverse consequences that can be precipitated by the rise in testosterone levels.

Tolerance and Side-Effects (Table 6)

In general the drug seems to be well tolerated. Compared to placebo, nilutamide given at a dose of 300 mg daily in surgically castrated patients did not show any differences in the incidence of adverse side-effects. The same was true when nilutamide was associated with GnRH analogues.
There is, however, one significant difference as the drug provokes visual disturbances in quite a proportion of patients. Delayed adaptation to darkness, especially after exposure to bright light, has been observed as the main side-effect in nearly all trials. While in treated patients there was a reported incidence of 27% (20% to 65% according to the different study groups), this effect has only been seen in about 4% of the patients on placebo [12,15,19-20]. Ophthalmological examination did not reveal any anatomical changes in the eye, although prolonged disturbance in darkness adaptation was measured in some patients. Interruption of therapy or dose reduction reverted the dark-adaptation time to normal. In some patients there was a spontaneous recovery despite continuation of treatment [11,19].
Gastrointestinal side-effects, mainly mild to moderate nausea and vomiting reported by about 12% of patients, are common in the initial weeks of therapy and most often disappear after the first month. They are seldom a motive to interrupt or postpone the treatment.
Transient hepatotoxicity, a shared feature of all antiandrogens, has been infrequently described with Anandron. Less than 1% of hepatitis has been reported in the treated groups, with recovery after discontinuation of therapy being the rule [1,14,15,20-22]. Spontaneously reversible increases in hepatic transaminases, generally occurring within the first 4 weeks of therapy, have been noted in up to 8% of nilutamide-treated patients.
Alcohol intolerance reactions similar to those described with disulfiram have been documented in about 5% of all patients treated with nilutamide [1,13,15].
Other less common side-effects such as pruritus, headache, vertigo and dizziness have been observed sporadically [15].
A more troublesome feature is the appearance in less than 2% of treated patients of an interstitial pneumonitis that can progress to pulmonary fibrosis [12,15]. In most cases it is, however, reversible on immediate cessation of nilutamide administration [24-26]. Akaza had to prematurely terminate a nilutamide study in Japan as 12.6% of his patients developed interstitial lung disease [4]. This complication has been mainly observed in Japan and much less in other trials worldwide.
Two other effects of androgen withdrawal, hot flushes and gynaecomastia, are commonly seen. In most studies comparing nilutamide versus placebo in combination with surgical or medical castration, their incidence was not significantly different [9,15,16]. When nilutamide was given as monotherapy hot flushes were reported in 53% of patients [1]. In this same study gynaecomastia was observed in 44% of men receiving nilutamide. In another trial combining nilutamide with a GnRH agonist, painful breast swelling was seen in 20% of patients [11].
A potentially beneficial effect is the favourable action the drug seems to exert on the plasma lipids with an increase in the proportion of HDL cholesterol [27].

Table 6. Most frequently occurring adverse events

	Castration* + Placebo N = 805	Castration* + Anandron N = 876
Hot flushes	36%	43%
Impaired adaption to darknesss	4%	27%
Nausea	5%	12%
Dizziness	4%	8%
Alcohol intolerance	2%	6%

* Either orchidectomy or LHRH agonist

In conclusion, it appears that the drug is well tolerated by the majority of patients. Compliance in nearly all trials as assessed by plasma drug assays was good. The safety profile is somewhat different from that of flutamide, with no diarrhoea, but with impaired adaption to darkness and the more serious but rare occurrence of interstitial pneumonitis.

What is the Place of Nilutamide in the Management of Prostatic Cancer?

Like the other specific antiandrogens, nilutamide, through its effect on the hypothalamic-pituitary-gonadal axis, increases LH and testosterone. Since the efficacy of monotherapy has not been investigated in large long-term comparative trials, it is difficult to state that monotherapy with nilutamide in patients with prostatic carcinoma is as beneficial as other treatments. Its essential advantage over conventional treatment is the possible maintenance of sexual function in a certain number of patients. This has also been reported with other pure antiandrogens and might improve the quality of life of those patients that are interested in preserving their sexual potency.
The association, however, of this drug with surgical or medical castration causes complete androgen blockade, resulting in an improvement of the efficacy over castration alone as regards metastatic pain, response to treatment, time to progression and thus quality of survival. Its long half-life offers the convenience of a once-daily dosage and the subsequent benefit for compliance. Furthermore, nilutamide is a pure antiandrogen devoid of any other hormonal activity. In the light of these advantages the safety profile seems to be quite acceptable.

Acknowledgement

The author is indebted to Dr A. de Géry and Dr M. Gaillard-Moguilewsky for their help in the preparation of this manuscript.

REFERENCES

1 Decensi AU, Boccardo F, Guarneri D et al: Monotherapy with nilutamide, a pure nonsteroidal antiandrogen, in untreated patients with metastatic carcinoma of the prostate. J Urol 1991 (146):377-381
2 Decensi AU, Torrisi K, Fontana V et al: Long term endocrine effects of administration of either a nonsteroidal antiandrogen or a luteinizing hormone-releasing hormone agonist in men with prostate cancer. Acta Endocrinol 1993 (129):315-321
3 Bertagna C, de Géry A, Hucher M, Francois JP, Zanirato J: Efficacy of the combination of Anandron (nilutamide) with orchidectomy in metastatic cancer. A metaanalysis of seven randomized double-blind trials (1191 patients). Br J Urol 1994 (in press)
4 Akaza H, Aso Y, Niijima T et al: Clinical study of RU 23908 (nilutamide) in prostatic cancer. Hinyokika Kiyo 1991 (37):407-420
5 Le Duc A, Arvis G, Ballanger R et al: Comparaison de l'efficacité du nilutamide (Anandron) à un placebo sur les douleurs des métastases osseuses de cancer de la prostate. Progrès en Urologie 1992 (suppl 2):24-30
6 Labrie F, Dupont A, Bélanger A et al: New approach in the treatment of prostate cancer: complete instead of partial withdrawal of androgens. Prostate 1983 (4):579-594
7 Labrie F, Dupont A, Bélanger A et al: Traitement anti-androgénique combiné dans l'adénocarcinome de la prostate: première application d'un nouveau principe thérapeutique efficace dans le cancer hormono-dépendant. Annales d'Urologie 1986 (20): 98-106
8 Kuhn J-M, Billebaud T, Navratil H et al: Prevention of the transient adverse effects of a gonadotrophin-releasing hormone analogue (buserelin) in metastatic prostate carcinoma by administration of an antiandrogen nilutamide. N Engl J Med 1989 (321): 413-418
9 Navratil H: Double blind study of Anandron versus placebo in stage D2 prostate cancer patients receiving buserelin: results on 49 cases from a multicentre study. In: Murphy G, Khoury S, Kuss P, Chatelain C and Denis L (eds) Prostatic Cancer. Part A. Alan R Liss, New York 1987 pp 401-410
10 Navratil H: Preliminary clinical evaluation of leuprolin acetate depot injection in France, in the management of prostatic cancer. J Internat Med Res 1990 (18 suppl 1):69-73
11 Migliari R, Scarpa RM, Campus G et al: Evaluation of efficacy and tolerability of nilutamide and buserelin in the treatment of advanced prostate cancer. Archivio Italiano di Urologia Andrologia 1991 (63): 147-153
12 Crawford ED, Smith Jr, Soloway MS et al: Treatment of stage D2 prostatic cancer with leuprolide and Anandron compared to leuprolide and placebo. In: Murphy G et al (eds) Recent Advances in Urological Cancers and Diagnosis and Treatment. Paris, 1990 pp 61-62
13 Brisset JM, Boccon-Gibod L, Botto H et al: Anandron (RU 23908) associated to surgical castration in previously untreated stage D prostate cancer. Part

A: Research, endocrine treatment and histopathology. Alan R Liss, New York 1987 pp 411-422

14 Namer M, Teubel J, Caby A et al: A ransomized double-blind study evaluating Anandron associated with orchiectomy in stage D prostate cancer. J Ster Biochem Mol Biol 1990 (37):909-915

15 Béland G, Elhilali M, Fradet Y et al: Total androgen ablation: Canadian experience. Urologic Clinics of North America 1991 (18):75-82

16 Janknegt RA, Abbou CC, Bartoletti R et al: Orchiectomy and nilutamide or placebo as treatment of metastatic prostatic cancer in a multinational double-blind randomized trial. J Urol 1993 (149):77-83

17 Smith JA, Crawford ED, Lange PH et al: PSA. Correlation with response and survival in advanced carcinoma of the prostate. In: Abstract book AUA San Antonio 1993 # 868

18 Abbou C, Brisset JM, Bracken B et al: Prostate specific antigen prognostic value for response to treatment in stage D2 prostate cancer patients: evaluation in a large study (457 patients) with central PSA assay. European Urology Xth EAU Congress, Genoa 22-25 July 1992, abstract # 267

19 Harnois C, Malenfant M, Dupont A, Labrie F: Ocular toxicity of anandron in patients treated for prostatic cancer. Br J Ophtalmol 1986 (70):471-473

20 Boccardo F, Decensi AU, Guarneri D et al: Anandron (RU 23908) in metastatic prostate cancer: Preliminary results of multicentric Italian study. Cancer Detect Prevent 1991 (15):501-503

21 Hammel P, Ducreux M, Bismuth E et al: Acute hepatitis related to the use of nilutamide (Anadron®). Gastroenterologie Clinique et Biologique 1991 (15): 557

22 Gomez JL, Dupont A, Cusan L et al: Simultaneous liver and lung toxicity related to the nonsteroidal antiandrogen nilutamide (Anandron): a case report. Am J Med 1992 (92):563-566

23 Seigneur J, Trechot PF, Hubert J: Pulmonary complications of hormone treatment in prostate carcinoma. Chest 1988 (93):1106

24 Pfitzenmeyer P, Foucher P, Piard F et al: Nilutamide pneumonitis: a report on 8 patients. Thorax 1992 (47):622-627

25 Jonville AP, Diot E, Dutertre JP, Autret E: Toxicité pulmonaire du nilutamide (Anadron®). Bilan Cooperatif des Centres Français de Pharmacovigilance. Therapie 1992 (47):393-397

26 Camus P, Coudert B, D'Athis P et al: Pharmacokinetics and metabolism of nilutamide in the isolated rat lung. J Pharmacol Exper Ther 1991 (259):1247-1255

27 Moorjani S, Dupont A, Labrie F et al: Increase in plasma high-density lipoprotein concentration following complete androgen blockage in men with prostatic carcinoma. Metabolism 1987 (36):244-250

28 Brisset JM: Nilutamide (Anandron®) in prostate cancer: Review of four clinical trials. In: Khoury S, Chatelain C, Denis L (eds) Urology. Prostate Cancer. Fiis et RGP, Paris 1990 pp 381-389

29 Du Plessis DDJ: Castration plus nilutamide vs castration plus placebo in advanced prostate cancer: a review. Urology 1991 (37 suppl 2):20-24

30 Knönagel H, Bolle JF, Hering F et al: Die Therapie des metastasierten Prostatakarzinoms durch Orchiektomie plus Anandron versus Orchiektomie plus Placebo. Erste Ergebnisse einer randomisierten Multizenterstudie. Helv Chir Acta 1989 (56):343-345

Indications for Antiandrogen Treatment in Prostate Cancer

Louis Denis

Oncological Centre Antwerp, Department of Urology, A.Z. Middelheim, Lindendreef 1, Antwerp 2020, Belgium

Steroidal Antiandrogens

The modern concept of antiandrogenic activity in prostate cancer has its origin in the development of cyproterone acetate (CPA) in 1962. Antiandrogens were first defined by Dorfman as substances that prevent androgens from expressing their activity at target sites. The inhibitory effect of these substances should be differentiated from that of substances decreasing the synthesis or release of gonadotrophins or inhibiting the biosynthesis and/or secretion of androgens [1]. This rather vague but accurate description was supported by the development of the receptor concept, according to which antiandrogens compete with androgens for the occupation of the nuclear receptor sites [2].

Ironically, the side effects of elegant animal experiments have revealed the pharmacological activity of CPA, which was conceived to be a potent hydroxyprogestogen. As a matter of fact, it is 3 times more potent than chlormadinone acetate (CMA) and 12 times more potent than medroxyprogesterone acetate (MPA). Both these drugs, as well as megoestrol acetate, another progestin with antiandrogenic activity, have been used in the treatment of metastatic prostate cancer.

It is interesting that all progestins have been observed to exert an agonistic effect on the androgen receptor, either by the anabolic properties of megoestrol acetate or by the steroid hormone withdrawal remission in patients with advanced hormone-refractory prostate cancer.

All these compounds have in common that they have a steroid structure and are provided with progestational activity causing antigonadotrophic effects (i.e., castration and impotence), and with antiandrogenic activity. In other words, these drugs have combined activity against prostate cancer and are accepted in monotherapy as well as in combination treatment.

Since the first clinical studies by Scott and Schirmer [3] it has been acknowledged that CPA is an effective treatment of prostate cancer at an oral dose of 3 x 100 mg tablets per day. The main cardiovascular side effects attributed to CPA are oedema and gynaecomastia, with no definite proof of increased cardiovascular death.

CPA has been combined with castration to evaluate the efficacy of this association. So far no advantage as regards progression or survival has been shown in two EORTC trials comparing this combination to orchidectomy or diethylstilboestrol (DES) 1 mg. We are also unaware as to whether responses can be obtained by giving CPA to patients with hormone-refractory prostate cancer [4]. CPA can be used, however, to suppress the clinical effects of the increase in serum testosterone (T) following a first injection of a luteotropic hormone releasing hormone (LHRH) agonist. The recommended timing, just as for DES, is one week before the initiation of LHRH-A therapy [5].

Of clinical use is the observation that hot flushes caused by castration can be prevented by CPA and megoestrol acetate. CPA can decrease the gynaecomastia induced by castration. There has been serious controversy as to the useful antiandrogenic action of CPA. This seems rather a theoretical problem since the main indication for prescribing non-steroidal antiandrogen monotherapy is the preservation of libido and potency, which excludes CPA in the

Table 1. Cyproterone Acetate (CPA)

Dose	50 mg tablets 3 x 2 per day
Side effects	Castration Gynaecomastia Cardiovascular Hepatic toxicity
Indications	Alternative to castration Prevent hot flushes Prevent LHRH-A flare-up

Table 2. Flutamide

Dose	250 mg tablets 3 x 1 per day
Side effects	Gynaecomastia Diarrhoea Nausea and vomiting Hepatic toxicity
Indications	Monotherapy: sex preservation MAB treatment Prevent LHRH-A flare-up

first place. Neumann states it clearly: "Non-steroidal antiandrogens are relatively more effective in castrated and androgen-replaced animals than CPA. In intact animals, CPA is much more active". The overall efficacy of CPA and flutamide in untreated patients with good prognostic factors is being evaluated in a prospective EORTC study. The clinical indications for CPA and its side effects are summarised in Table 1.

Non-Steroidal Antiandrogens

Flutamide

A number of animal experiments have demonstrated the antiandrogenic activity of flutamide (SCH 13521) in various species [6]. It is a substituted anilide with a half-life of 8 hours in men; its major metabolite, hydroxyflutamide, is responsible for most of the antiandrogenic activity. Because of its anilide structure, methaemoglobin studies were performed in a number of species, among which only the cat proved to be sensitive.

Administration of flutamide increases the levels of LH, resulting in raised serum testosterone (T) and oestrogen (E) levels that induce breast pain and gynaecomastia in males. These increases are dose related.

Based on animal experiments and patient responses to 375 mg or 1,500 mg per day, the conventional dose has been estimated to be 250 mg tid per os [7]. The clinical indications, side effects and dose of flutamide are presented in Table 2.

A number of uncontrolled phase II studies have been conducted on the use of flutamide as monotherapy. Objective and subjective responses of variable duration in hormone-naive or hormone-refractory patients have been observed [8,9]. In small randomised trials similar efficacy was shown for flutamide 750 mg per day and DES 1 or 3 mg per day and oestramustine phosphate in untreated patients with prostate cancer. Flutamide may cause fewer cardiovascular complications and its side effects include nausea and diarrhoea, hepatic toxicity and gynaecomastia. Its main appeal is the preservation of libido and potency, a factor likely to improve quality of life in selected patients. Flushing is not associated with monotherapy, but may occur in half of the patients treated with flutamide and medical or surgical castration.

Prout et al. showed a better and longer progression-free response in untreated patients related to the total tumour burden [9]. It is not surprising that the response is usually limited and short in hormone-refractory patients. Nevertheless, a positive response was obtained in 31% of patients in whom CPA in combination treatment was replaced by flutamide, including 58% of those with node-positive disease [10]. The results of combination treatment or maximal androgen blockade (MAB) are described in detail by Labrie et al. in this volume.

The subject of MAB treatment is still controversial. Studies of MAB versus castration only are inconclusive when viewed collectively, although the mature and largest trials showed an advantage for MAB. The remaining studies have insufficient power to reveal the extent of its effect. No study shows MAB to be inferior to surgical or medical castration alone. The INT 0105 trial involving 1,200 patients in progress may permit firmer conclusions. Meanwhile we have to live with a rather modest overall survival and a more impressive progression-free survival for patients treated with MAB [11].

A quite singular clinical scenario has recently gained the spotlight: "The flutamide withdrawal syndrome". It has been observed that the nuclear receptors of patients undergoing hormonal treatment (including oestrogens and progestins) adapted to joint mutation in the hormone binding domain, which changes the action from antagonist to agonist. The positive effects of flutamide withdrawal in progressing patients not only caused remarkable PSA decreases but also clinical responses in measurable disease [12]. Therefore, flutamide or steroid hormone withdrawal appears to be the first therapeutic choice in patients progressing after a positive response to MAB treatment.

Nilutamide

Nilutamide (RU 23908) is a non-steroidal antiandrogen which interacts with the androgen receptor but not with other steroid hormone receptors. *In vitro* studies have demonstrated interaction with the androgen receptor to form a low-affinity, unstable complex that shows little recovery in the nucleus and prevents interaction by the endogenous androgens. It has also been demonstrated that high doses may inhibit enzyme pathways in testosterone biosynthesis. Interaction of nilutamide in both peripheral and central target organs causes increases in LH and testosterone [13].

In vitro and *in vivo* studies on cell lines and animal models have shown excellent antiandrogenic results in castrated animals but a lack of total inhibition in intact animals. All further research focussed on a potentiating effect of castration by nilutamide. Apart from dose-related anaemia, no toxicity was observed in animal experiments.

Studies in healthy males showed a mean half-life of 45 hours. This allows once-daily administration of 300 mg to reach a steady state after 2 weeks.

A few trials used nilutamide as monotherapy in M1 prostate cancer patients. Response rates of 38.5% in untreated patients and of 5.5% in relapsed patients were reported. The side effects included delayed visual adaptation to darkness, nausea, interstitial pneumonitis and alcohol intolerance. Half of the potent patients reported preservation of libido and potency [14].

Table 3. Nilutamide

Dose	300 mg tablet once daily for 1 month then 150 mg
Side effects	Gynaecomastia Visual dark adaptation Nausea and vomiting Hepatic toxicity Alcohol intolerance Interstitial pneumonitis
Indications	Monotherapy: Sex preservation MAB treatment Prevent LHRH-A flare-up

A series of 7 randomised trials using nilutamide with orchidectomy as MAB treatment versus orchidectomy and placebo were analysed in an overview including 1,191 patients [15]. All response rates were significantly better for the MAB treatment while disease progression was statistically lower (16% reduction), with a downward trend in survival. Nilutamide combined with LHRH-A provided better responses and a small difference in median time to progression (2.1 months) [16]. Similar studies have provided sufficient support for the role of nilutamide in preventing the disease flare induced by the initial injection of LHRH-A.

Dose ranging studies settled on 300 mg as a single daily dose for one month and 150 mg thereafter as effective treatment. The dose, reported side effects and indications are presented in Table 3.

Bicalutamide

This compound (ICI 176334) was identified for development as a non-steroidal antiandrogen that would be peripherally selective, i.e., the lack of action at the hypothalamic-pituitary gonadal axis would prevent a secondary LH and T rise [17].

The promising peripheral selectivity in mature male rats is due to poor penetration of the drug through the blood-brain barrier and could not be reproduced in other species, including man. The affinity for binding to the androgen receptor in rat, dog and human prostate is low compared to the natural ligand but still 4 times higher in the rat and 50 times higher in the dog than with hydroxyflutamide.

Bicalutamide was effective in reducing Dunning R 3227 H tumours. In all preclinical studies bicalutamide was well tolerated, with no secondary effects except on the dog's heart rate at high doses.
With daily doses of 50 mg, steady-state plasma concentrations are registered after several weeks. The half-life of the drug is approximately 6 days, making it suitable for once-daily treatment. The lack of toxicity, the once-daily dose and the reported efficacy led to a number of phase II and phase III trials using bicalutamide at different doses as monotherapy and as part of MAB treatment. These clinical studies were preceded by dose finding studies evaluating a drop of 50% in patients with prostate cancer in whom prostatic acid phosphatase serum levels were raised to twice their normal values. At daily doses of 10, 30 and 50 mg decreases of this range were noted in 33%, 53% and 83% of treated patients. Based on these results and on the absence of any toxic effects, the 50 mg dose was chosen as the standard in the first randomised studies [18].
The availability of prostate specific antigen (PSA) as a secondary surrogate endpoint prompted further dose ranging studies to evaluate the dose-related safety and the increasing therapeutic response. The effects for a range of doses up to 150 mg are shown in Table 4 [19].
The feared secondary increase in LH and T was observed. The T serum levels showed an approximately 60% rise with respect to pretreatment levels but controls of up to 3 years have demonstrated that there is a plateau after 1 year without further increases [20].
A first open, multicentre study focussed on the safety and efficacy of a once daily dose of 50 mg. Objective responses were observed in 70% of 150 patients and 40% had a 90% PSA decrease or normalisation. Extent of disease was a significant predictor of response. Gynaecomastia occurred in 60% of the patients, diarrhoea in 5%. The conclusion was that trials evaluating higher doses as monotherapy, as well as MAB treatment, were recommended [21].
This prophetic conclusion was tested in 3 randomised, controlled trials comparing 50 mg of bicalutamide to either surgical or medical castration (LHRH-A) or bilateral orchidectomy. The results, based on an analysis of over 1,000 patients with objective and subjective criteria, favoured castration over 50 mg of bicalutamide. The difference was not only a lower median drop in PSA (87% vs 97%) but a $p > 0.001$ difference in time to treatment failure and median survival. Comparison of the pharmacological effects showed more gynaecomastia, better preservation of sexual functioning and less hot flushing in patients on the drug. It was recommended to use higher doses of bicalutamide since similar adverse events were noted in studies with doses up to 150 mg per day [22]. This dose was tested in 2 randomised trials involving 1,453 patients with M1 or Mo prostate cancer. An interim analysis of the M1 patients showed castration to yield better results than bicalutamide ($p = 0.002$), while the hazard ratio was well balanced in the Mo patients with a trend towards an advantage for the drug-treated patients. The study coordinators terminated the M1 trial. This situation prompted renewed interest in higher doses of up to 450 mg a day, although pharmacokinetic evaluation studies suggested no major additional benefit could be expected of doses over 200 mg per day.
The incidence of adverse effects due to pharmacological action showed again the gynaecomastia vs hot flushes tendency. Secondary responses after the flutamide withdrawal syndrome have been described and should be carefully evaluated.

Table 4. Percentage of PSA decline and normalisation at 3 months*

	10 mg	30 mg	50 mg	100 mg	150 mg	CAS
% PSA decline	57	73	90	97	97	97
% PSA normalisation			22	25	62	40

* adapted from Tables 2 and 3 [19]

Table 5. Bicalutamide

Dose	Monotherapy 150 mg per day and up MAB 50 mg per day
Side effects	Gynaecomastia Diarrhoea Hepatotoxicity
Indications	Monotherapy: sex preservation MAB treatment Prevent LHRH-A flare-up

Bicalutamide has been evaluated in MAB treatment in 813 patients in a 2 x 2 factorial design comparing flutamide, goserelin acetate and leuprolide acetate. With a median follow-up of 49 weeks, time to treatment failure was significantly better for the bicalutamide arm ($p = 0.006$). As regards the adverse events, diarrhoea was recorded in 10% of the bicalutamide arm leading to withdrawal in 0.5%, compared to 24% of the flutamide arm leading to withdrawal in 6.1% of the patients ($p = 0.001$) [23].
We conclude that bicalutamide is an efficacious, well tolerated compound, to be used in monotherapy as clinical research in Mo prostate cancer, and in combination to prevent flare-up or as MAB treatment. The usual dose, adverse events and indications are presented in Table 5.

Use of the Antiandrogens in Endocrine Treatment

The standard treatment for symptomatic metastatic disease is to ablate or block the androgens that stimulate the prostate cancer cells. No other therapy matches the number of subjective and objective responses.
The obvious question "Is there a best primary hormonal treatment?" can be answered by looking at the array of current endocrine treatments in general use as shown in Table 6.
Surgical castration is by far the most cost-effective treatment; however, considering that 15% to 30% of the treated patients do not respond to hormone withdrawal, it is no surprise that more and more patients opt for reversible medical castration by LHRH-A. There is consensus that the initial LHRH-A produces a rise in testosterone that may cause clinical harm by overstimulation of the tumour, especially in patients with hydronephrosis, widespread metastatic disease or threatening spinal cord compression.

Table 6. Array of current first-line endocrine treatments utilised in daily practice to palliate prostate cancer

Androgen Withdrawal	
1. Surgical castration:	Bilateral orchidectomy Subcapsular orchidectomy Subepididymal orchidectomy
2. Medical castration:	Oestrogens Diethylstilboestrol 1-3 mg/day Polyoestradiol phosphate i.m. 160 mg/month Estramustine phosphate 560 mg/day
LHRH-A:	Depot preparations
Androgen Blockade	
Antiandrogens*	Cyproterone acetate 300 mg/day Flutamide 750 mg/day* Nilutamide 300 mg/day* Bicalutamide 150 mg/day
Combination Treatment	
Maximal Androgen Blockade	LHRH-A - antiandrogen Castration - antiandrogen

* monotherapy of non-steroidal antiandrogens is clinical research

It is fair to state that all antiandrogens listed can prevent this clinical flare phenomenon by prior administration. The usual dose of the antiandrogen is sufficient (see Table 6) and should be continued for 2 weeks. This is the first and uncontested indication for the use of antiandrogens in oncological practice.

Monotherapy resulting in castrate T levels is the therapeutic effect of the steroid antiandrogens. They can be used as an alternative to surgical or LHRH-A castration, keeping in mind that the progestins cause cardiovascular toxicity, especially in patients with cardiovascular disease. Treatment with non-steroidal antiandrogens, on the other hand, gives rise to partially potency-sparing serum T, resulting in a sense of general well-being for the treated male. This is particularly appealing to the potent male and discussing his palliative treatment and the preservation of sexual function guides the patient's preference to non-steroidal antiandrogens. Breast tenderness and gynaecomastia, rather common side effects of this type of monotherapy, should be discussed with the patient.

Unfortunately, we have no scientific proof that an antiandrogen is equivalent to other types of endocrine treatment, in particular castration. There is consensus that the response rates are lower and time to progression is shorter for any of the non-steroidal antiandrogens as compared to castration. Bicalutamide at 150 mg per day produced PSA decreases and normalisation equivalent to castration but proved inferior in M1 disease. The finding that the trends in Mo disease were in favour of bicalutamide reminds us of the observation of Prout [8] and Soloway [21] that the extent of disease determines response and duration of response. This leaves us with a viable motive for continuing our monotherapy trials, but focussed on the early stages of the disease.

Monotherapy with non-steroidal antiandrogens, a treatment aimed at blocking both testicular and adrenal androgens, still offers hope for refinement of the compounds or increasing or facilitating the blockade by adding atoxic 5-alpha-reductase blockers or, as seen, by starting treatment in the earliest stages of the disease.

Preserving sexual potency in well informed patients is the second indication for antiandrogens in the endocrine treatment of prostate cancer. It is advised to monitor these patients carefully with attention to detail and to make common-sense decisions. A satisfied patient with a normalised PSA has a long way to go.

Is there a best antiandrogen? Although the blocking effect is dose dependent, the toxicity is a limitation. The safety profile of bicalutamide seems convincing even at the 150 mg per day dose. The reported side effects of the three non-steroidal antiandrogens are listed in Table 7.

The third indication to improve treatment efficacy is still controversial and involves the added effect of the antiandrogen to castration. Considering that the survival gain is modest but the time to progression rather important, we have to settle for patient selection. Advantages, especially in response and time to progression, have invariably been reported for flutamide and nilutamide combinations.

The use of the steroidal antiandrogens in MAB treatment has to be discouraged since we have never seen results in favour of the combination with these compounds. They do carry some non-lethal cardiovascular toxicity and their pharmacotherapeutic profile is not needed in the combination.

Table 7. Side effects reported for the three antiandrogens in the reported dosages
The side effects are dose dependent

Side effects	Flutamide	Nilutamide	Bicalutamide
Gynaecomastia	+	+	+
Diarrhoea	++	-	±
Nausea	+	+	-
Liver tests	+	±	-
Visual adaptation	-	+	-
Lung toxicity	-	+	-
Alcohol intolerance	-	+	-

Table 8. Clinical use of steroidal and non-steroidal antiandrogens

	STEROIDAL ANTIANDROGENS
Advanced cancer	Alternative to castration Prevention of flare-up by LHRH-A Hot flushes
	NON-STEROIDAL ANTIANDROGENS
Advanced cancer	Monotherapy MAB treatment Monotherapy and 5-alpha-reductase Prevention of flare-up by LHRH-A Hormone-refractory disease Replacement of compounds having become agonists over time
Early cancer	Debulking before surgery/radiotherapy Adjuvant after radical surgery

In an ongoing randomised trial the newcomer bicalutamide in combination with LHRH-A gave significantly better results ($p = 0.006$) in time to treatment failure. Diarrhoea proved to be the main adverse effect, leading to withdrawal of 0.5% of the patients (compared to 6.1% with flutamide). Assessment of survival requires additional follow-up.

We believe that the third indication for the use of non-steroidal antiandrogens lies in the added blocking of the adrenal androgens after surgical or medical castration.

From the controversy surrounding the meta-analysis of 23 studies involving MAB treatment, it is clear that patients with poor prognostic factors have no chance nor time to profit from the intended effect. Once again, however, there is a trend towards better responses and longer progression-free survival in almost all trials evaluating the combination, along with a gain in survival in some studies. It is difficult to accept the controversy since it has been agreed and confirmed that antiandrogens induce secondary remissions in 7% to 30% of patients with progression of disease after remission on primary endocrine treatment. With MAB treatment, one simply brings this modest advantage upfront in the hope that a smaller tumour burden will respond better and longer. The 1,200 patient NCI 0115 study will provide a definite answer to this question.

Promiscuity of the androgen receptors, probably due to the development of mutations affecting gene activation that turns antiandrogenic action into agonistic activity, has been reported for a number of compounds including steroid hormones such as oestrogens and hydrocortisone. Based on these observations, it has become clear that in prostate cancer patients in progression after earlier remissions a discontinuation of these compounds is warranted prior to the use of more toxic chemotherapy. The field of secondary hormonal treatment is wide open to further observations and more extensive research.

This brings us to the fourth indication for the use of antiandrogens, namely as first-line therapy in relapsed patients, or to replace a mismatch of an androgen receptor by another antiandrogen.

In conclusion, we can state that the development of the non-steroidal antiandrogens has introduced a new concept in our therapeutic strategy for prostate cancer that is still evolving. Some extra comfort and maybe life are appreciated by the patients, but their strongest preference is for monotherapy with preservation of sexuality, especially among younger patients.

Steroidal and non-steroidal antiandrogens are very different drugs which merit use in the clinical settings presented in Table 8. It is vital to proceed in an orderly manner, with the support of randomised trials if possible, and if not, with demonstration data of good quality. The urologists carry the burden of finding appropriate answers to these unresolved questions.

REFERENCES

1 Dorfman RI: Anti-androgenic substances. In: Dorfman RI (ed) Methods in Hormone Research, Vol. II. Academic Press, New York, London 1962 pp 315-323

2 Jensen EV, Jacobson HI: Basic guides to the mechanism of estrogen action. Recent Progr Horm Res 1962 (18):387

3 Scott WW, Schirmer HK: A new oral progestational steroid effective in treating prostatic cancer. Trans Am Assoc Genito-Urin Surg 1966 (58):54-62

4 Denis L, Murphy GP: Overview of phase III trials on combined androgen treatment in patients with metastatic prostate cancer. Cancer 1993 (72):3888-3895

5 Boccon-Gibod L, Laudat MH, Dugue MA, Steg A: Cyproterone acetate lead-in prevents initial rise of serum testosterone induced by LHRH analogs in the treatment of metastatic carcinoma of the prostate. Eur Urol 1986 (12):400-402

6 Neri RO, Florence K, Koziol P, Van Cleave S: A biological profile of a nonsteroidal antiandrogen, SCH 13521 (4'-nitro-3'-trifluoromethylisobutyranilide). Endocrinology 1972 (91):427-437

7 Prout GRP et al: Prostatic cancer and SCH 13521. II. Histological alterations and the pituitary gonadal axis. J Urol 1974 (113):834

8 Prout GR Jr, Keating MA, Griffin PP, Schiff SF: Long-term experience with flutamide in patients with prostatic carcinoma. Urology 1989 (34):37-45

9 Sogani PC, Vagaiwala MR, Whitmore WF Jr: Experience with flutamide in patients with advanced prostatic cancer without prior endocrine therapy. Cancer 1984 (54):744

10 Brogden RN, Chrisp P: Flutamide: A review of its pharmacodynamic and pharmacokinetic properties, and therapeutic use in advanced prostatic cancer. Drugs & Aging 1991 (1):104-115

11 Denis L: Maximal androgen blockade in prostate cancer: A theory to put into practice? Br J Urol 1995 (submitted)

12 Scher HI, Kelly WK: Flutamide withdrawal syndrome: Its impact on clinical trials in hormone refractory prostate cancer. J Clin Oncol 1993 (11):1566-1572

13 Ojasoo T: Nilutamide. Drugs of the Future 1987 (12): 763-770

14 Decensi AU, Boccardo F, Guarneri D et al: Monotherapy with nilutamide, a pure nonsteroidal anti-androgen, in untreated patients with metastatic carcinoma of the prostate. J Urol 1991 (146):377-381

15 Bertagna C, de Géry A, Hucher M, Francois JP, Zanirato J: Efficacy of the combination of Anandron (nilutamide) with orchidectomy in metastatic cancer. A metaanalysis of seven randomized double-blind trials (1,191 patients). Br J Urol 1994 (73):396-402

16 Crawford ED, Smith Jr, Soloway MS et al: Treatment of stage D2 prostatic cancer with leuprolide and Anandron compared to leuprolide and placebo. In: Murphy G et al (eds) Recent Advances in Urological Cancers and Diagnosis and Treatment. SCI, Paris 1990 pp 61-62

17 Furr BJA, Valcaccia B, Curry B, Woodburn JR, Chesterson G, Tucker H: ICI 176334: a novel nonsteroidal peripherally selective antiandrogen. J Endocrinol 1987 (113):7-9

18 Newling DWW: The response of advanced prostate cancer to a new non-steroidal anti-androgen: Results of a multicenter open phase II study of Casodex. Eur Urol 1990 (19):18-21

19 Blackledge G: Casodex - Mechanisms of action and opportunities for usage. Cancer 1993 (72):3830-3833

20 Mahler Ch, Van Cangh P, Bouffioux Ch, Keuppens F, Coeck C, Ongena P, Denis L: Endocrine effects of Casodex R, a new non-steroidal anti-androgen. In: Murphy G, Khoury S, Chatelain C, Denis L (eds) Proceedings of the Second International Symposium on Recent Advances in Urological Cancers: Diagnosis and Treatment. Wiley-Liss, New York 1991 pp 42-45

21 Soloway MS: Early clinical trials of bicalutamide as monotherapy for prostate cancer (phase II). Urology 1995 (submitted)

22 Kaisary AV: Current clinical studies with a new nonsteroidal antiandrogen, Casodex. The Prostate 1994 (5):27-33

23 Schellhammer P, Sharifi R, Block N, Soloway M, Venner P, Patterson AL, Sarosdy M, Jones J, Kolvenbag G for the Casodex Combination Study Group: Casodex R in combination therapy: A comparison with flutamide in patients with untreated metastatic prostate cancer. AUA Proceedings 1995

GPSR Compliance
The European Union's (EU) General Product Safety Regulation (GPSR) is a set of rules that requires consumer products to be safe and our obligations to ensure this.

If you have any concerns about our products, you can contact us on

ProductSafety@springernature.com

In case Publisher is established outside the EU, the EU authorized representative is:

Springer Nature Customer Service Center GmbH
Europaplatz 3
69115 Heidelberg, Germany

www.ingramcontent.com/pod-product-compliance
Lightning Source LLC
Chambersburg PA
CBHW061220240926
51846CB00006B/1291
9783642457470